Banned Drugs Versus Balanced Diet

"Performance in food as opposed to drug use/misuse/abuse"

Written
By

Alli-Balogun Alli-Baba

Co-ordinator
Parents and Athletes against Drugs in Sports
P.A.A.D.S
Since 1992
"Towards a Sustainable and predictable Healthy Life style!

Bloomington, IN 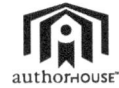 Milton Keynes, UK

authorHOUSE

AuthorHouse™
1663 Liberty Drive, Suite 200
Bloomington, IN 47403
www.authorhouse.com
Phone: 1-800-839-8640

AuthorHouse™ UK Ltd.
500 Avebury Boulevard
Central Milton Keynes, MK9 2BE
www.authorhouse.co.uk
Phone: 08001974150

This book is a work of non-fiction. Unless otherwise noted, the author and the publisher make no explicit guarantees as to the accuracy of the information contained in this book and in some cases, names of people and places have been altered to protect their privacy.

First published by AuthorHouse 3/1/2006

ISBN: 1-4208-8694-0 (sc)

Printed in the United States of America
Bloomington, Indiana

This book is printed on acid-free paper.

The secret is figuring out exactly what to eat and how to appropriately Combine diet and not banned drugs to achieve your objectives.

A Problem known......
Is Half Solved?
Banned Drugs versus Balanced Diet
A
Drug
Use/misuse/abuse
In
Sports
Cathartic book.

Banned Drugs versus Balanced Diet
(here on referred to as Bd versus Bd within the text)

Together we can make a difference; in the war against performance enhancing drugs in sport. In order to make such a prophecy come about, kindly make Bd versus Bd available to athletes and coaches. We also encourage fellow physical/health educators and enthusiasts to assist in this campaign by promoting and distributing this nutritional book within sport associations, clubs, training camps and gyms, both before, during and after championships.

Play your part in the war against drug use/misuse/abuse in competitive sport. This will help towards eliminating drugs in sport before it is too late.

Dedicated:

To

All competitive athletes that derive their energy to compete naturally from
balanced diet as* opposed to *banned drugs

"To balance your training and performance, you need a balanced diet and not

banned drugs"

YOU WILL BE HELD RESPONSIBLE

Warning

- *Do not wreck your sports career and bring shame on yourself, your family and friends by using/misusing/abusing banned drugs.*
- *Stay away from those who sell drugs because it is you in particular and not them that will suffer when you are caught.*
- *If you have proof, kindly report the drug sellers to the nearest anti-doping or law enforcement officer.*

IF IN DOUBT LEAVE IT OUT!

INTRODUCTION

The basic principle behind the book "Banned Drugs versus Balanced Diet" is to advise athletes on what they actually need and want from diet and nutrition. It is especially aimed at those in the minority who do not want to use/misuse/abuse anabolic-androgenic steroids and other toxic chemicals in the pursuance of medals. By the same token, we are interested in providing an effective and proven alternative to performance enhancing drugs through excellent dietary tips. This is to ensure that all sportsmen and women are on track to success, whilst being virtually 99% pure and natural.

This superbly organised diet book was written primarily to address all diet and nutrition related problems. We are sure that half truths will immediately start to disintegrate once athletes can access this book. The simple reason is that we will openly through this medium, explain to athletes what food is, how it works and functions, how it can be used effectively to ensure that their body mechanisms operate at full capacity.

Note, a *body operating at full health capacity means two things: -*

i) The potential for efficient performance and increased strength generating capability is optimised.

ii) The internal resistance to infection, diseases, stamina, recuperation and proper relaxation is accelerated.

Furthermore, a lot of in-depth research and analysis from every pragmatic approach went into Bd versus Bd at every level of its production that critically confirms to us the saying:

i) "What you eat is what you are".

ii) "Sports performance is in food and not in enhancing drugs"

iii) "The most intensive training is wasted without a proper balanced diet"- drawn from protein, carbohydrate, fat, vitamins, minerals and comprehensively reviewed dietary food supplementation"

Again, we advise athletes to start eating *"Close to nature"* in order to enjoy the true reward of advanced nutrition, compared to the zig – zag results of various "stacked" drugs, which bring no true or lasting benefit. In conclusion, it is intended that Bd versus Bd, will find a worthy place in the hearts of coaches, sport administrators, team managers, athlete's representatives, physical and health educators and the athletes for whom the book was primarily written......

ACKNOWLEDGEMENT

The author of Banned Drugs versus Balanced Diet would not have been able to present his view and findings so carefully with clear objectives without your outstanding support.

The book also provides:

1. A rewarding alternative to drug use/misuse/abuse among sportsmen and women.

2. Sound evidence that diet and nutrition is the make-or-break component of sports-building success.

3. A detailed account of everything needed in order to consistently optimize the progress of sportsmen and women

Organization:

- Hem-ufit Research/Verification Institution

- World Anti - Doping Agency (WADA)

- English institute of sports (EIS)

- Nigeria institute of sports (NIS)

- UK Sports

Specialized Individuals:

- **Dave Orshi** – Head of research (*P.A.A.D.S)*
- **Aliyu Jubril** – administration/*research team (P.A.A.D.S)*
- **Romilla Jones** – Copyeditor
- **Jimmy Curmning** - Sports psychologist
  Sports ace limited U.K.

We acknowledge the numerous academic and scientific sources of this text, and if due credit has not been given in footnotes or in any instance; forbearance is requested as most of the content has been culled from various diversified sources even when source material has been accessible.

FORWARD

Transparency and fair-play which are the corner stones of sport have been undermined by the senseless use/misuse/abuse of various performance enhancing drugs. We are now in a situation where drugs and sport often seem to go together like "fish and chips". It has become clearer at every level that several athletes have emerged as the alleged products of not just of talent, skills and perseverance but of various banned substances that contravene the ethics of both sport and medical science.

It is shameful to see athletes dying gradually in the pursuance of medals especially when this is preventable. The current big question is whether pharmaceutical drugs have positively or negatively revolutionized sport. As a former athlete and now a physical and health enthusiast, all I can say is that; they have done more harm and will continue to do more harm than good. Eventually, many athletes did not *get what they paid for, but paid dearly for what they got"*.

Competing with an unfair advantage is unsportsmanlike and no athlete should feel any pride or superiority towards fellow competitors from a victory achieved through doping. For this and many other reasons, is why we are launching this moral crusade to fight the scourge of drugs, a pandemic that is gradually destroying the essence of sport and threatens to devastate it's entire foundation. I am sure that no one will dispute my harrowing description of the human tragedy unfolding before us.

The book *"Banned Drugs versus Balanced Diet"* was written with a strict policy. That is to close loopholes, redirect the mind and to change the perception of the athletes and coaches; to also ensure that all stakeholders in sport accept that diet and nutrition are the alpha and omega of sport performance.

Our effort includes:-

- An extensive relationship with dietician and nutritionist

- The gathering of information from various cutting edge scientists in the sport and nutrition arena.

- Ensuring that any statement provided within this book will be of benefit to all our intended targets.

Since the administration of substances from prohibited classes of pharmacological agents, and/or the use of various prohibited methods among many athletes has continued unabated, it is my hope that the book Bd versus Bd will foster the correct attitude among the athletes. It is also my hope that it will restore confidence and integrity in the performance of worthy winners and eradicate the false belief that record breaking performances are an indication of the use/misuse/abuse drugs.

Dave Orshi
President
Parents and Athletes against Drugs in Sports (PAADS)

CONTENTS

Chapter One
EAT PROTEIN AND GROW FOR IT!

In sport and as well as in life in general, all types of physiological processes relating to energy, recovery, muscle strength gain, as well as mood and brain function are closely and directly linked to amino acids. The production of hormones, repair of skin, nails and hair are best taken care of when an abundance of amino acids and not anabolic-androgenic steroids are available in the body system.

Note: Amino acid is not a protein, but when a number of them clinically united become or form a protein.

Amino acids are the building blocks of protein and are so important that without sufficient amounts, your body will catabolise muscle tissue to derive what it needs. There may be from two to four hundred or more amino acids in a given protein and for you to achieve or sustain a reasonable amino acid profile throughout the day, you must consume a good variety of protein sources. These should include meat, soya, dairy and combinations of non-animal foods. This is simply to ensure that the best and most complete amino profile is entering your system.

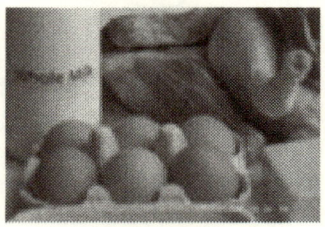

Animal protein is generally indispensable

We keep on and on wondering why so many athletes know so little about the major sources of amino acids, and significantly the importance of protein. This problem must be solved if a sports dream will ever come true, especially now that nothing less than optimal performance is a must for all competing athletes.

Note: Plants are able to build up or synthesize protein; animals including man cannot do this. They therefore must eat plants or animals that have already preyed upon plants to obtain their protein.

SIGNIFICANCE OF PROTEIN

Protein is not a wonder drug, but it will make the difference between everything working and everything not working. Protein should be considered as an essential basis for whatever sport you are competing in. Without sufficient or additional protein intake, you will not have adequate energy reserves to fuel the muscle you so badly need for maximum performance. In short, *"protein is the difference between success and failure"* Whatever sport you are doing, you are using your muscles. Without muscles you cannot run, walk, swim or jump, not to mention that of lifting weights in the gym.

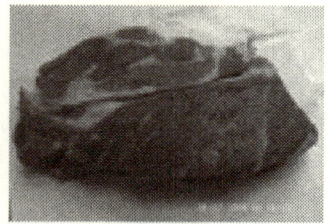

Red meats provide good source of protein

This statement is necessary because most tennis, cyclist, rugby players, or those in martial arts and so on, think they do not need both essential and non-essential protein to achieve an optimum performance. This notion is quite unrealistic.

Note: In the interest of health and performance, start giving your body and soul the extra protein it so badly needs now and I can assure you that in the nearest future you will reap the benefits.

All reliable evidence and research shows that your body is in constant demand of protein turnover 24 hours a day. Whether you train or not, your body requires a constant supply of protein to fuel virtually all the metabolic processes required for general health. Now imagine adding vigorous and rigorous training to this equation and for sure, the demand for protein by your body will definitely skyrocket!

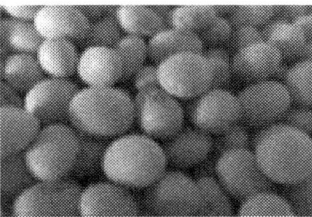

Soybeans, a good source of plant protein

Research reveals that many of our brothers and sisters in sport have been indoctrinated by inaccurate books, magazine articles and naive food supplement companies, persuading them that carbohydrates are the *"be all and end all"* and that they do not have much need for protein. Fellow athletes, if you are training 3-5 times per week or more; you are going to need 0.60 – 1.00 grams per pound of body weight or about 25% - 35% of total daily calories. Anything less than this, then you might as well stop aspiring to become a champion, pack up and go for a picnic!

Eating too little protein however, will adversely limit your strength level and stamina, weaken your immunological status and make you susceptible to an array of symptoms associated with a poor diet.

Note: A potion of fish weighing 31.25 grams contains approximately 7.6 grams of protein, equal to about 30 calories from protein.

(7.6 x 4 = 30.4) calories per gram = 4.

On a daily basis, your protein intake should consist of food with first class sources or protein of the highest nutritional value. Protein that should be eaten daily includes milk, eggs, meat, fish and cheese. These are sources of first class protein and are of the highest nutritional value and are so necessary for the body system to function in the

- Production of cells and hormones

- Boosting the immune system

- Promoting neurotransmitter activity

In any case, protein consumption should be the number one nutritional concern for any athlete. It is the major determining factor in the result you get from the hours you spend sweating it out in your quest to be a champion. It should be clear at this stage that life is impossible without protein. The physiological basis of life is largely made up of protein and not anabolic –androgenic chemicals

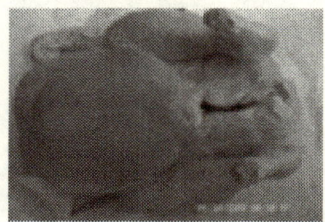

Poultry meat, an excellent source of animal protein

MAJOR SOURCES OF AMINO ACID

As many as 23 amino acids are the "molecular building blocks" of proteins according to the accepted clarification. (8) Eight are termed *"Essential or indispensable"*. These are amino acids that your body cannot manufacture on its own, or produce sufficiently to keep the system functioning smoothly and properly, and are called essential Amino acids. These (8) Eight must be consumed through various food sources.

Isoleucine	Lysine
Ieucine	Methionine
Valine	Phenylalanine
Tryptophan	Threonine

Conditionally essential or important Amino acids - as the name implies. These may be important or not, and will solely depend on the kind and type of event or activities that the athletes is involved in. For example, if the supply of essential amino acids in your diet is limited as a result of an intense training regimen, other amino acids can become essential in order to supplement the deficit.

Arginine	Histidine
Cystenine	Proline
Cystine	Tyrosine
Clutamine	

Non-essential, dispensable amino acids, conditionally indispensable – These are amino acids which your body can synthesize from other sources, such as fat or carbohydrate. They are non-essential and will remain so because you do not have to concern yourself about consuming foods high in these aminos.

Alanine	Glutamic acid
Asparagine	Glycine
Aspartic acid	Serine.

AMINO ACID GUIDE

INDISPENSABLE AMINO ACIDS

Indispensable amino acids, also called essential amino acids must be supplied to the body from good food sources.

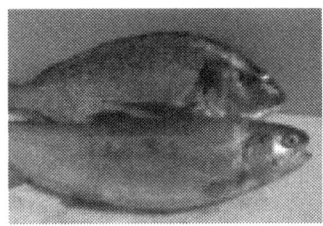

Fish provides a good source of protein (indispensable)

ISOLEUCINE

- A branched - chain amino acid, readily taken up and used for energy by muscle tissue

- Used to prevent muscle wasting in debilitated individuals

- Essential in the formation of haemoglobin

IEUCINE

- A branched – chain amino acid used as a source of energy

- Helps reduce muscle protein breakdown

- Modulates the uptake of neurotransmitter precursors by the brain as well as stimulating the release of adrenaline, which will inhibit the passage of pain signals to the nervous system.

- Promotes the healing of skin and the repairs broken bone

VALINE

- A branched – chain amino acid

- Not processed by the liver but actively taken up by muscle

- Influences the brain uptake of other neurotransmitter precursors *(tryptophan, phenylalanine and tyrosine)*.

TRYPTHOPHAN

- Helps athletes to maintain concentration and focus

- Ensures good mood and calmness required for performance

- Helps the brain to function properly *(Serotonin production)* -a chemical in the brain.

LYSINE

- Low levels can slow protein synthesis, affecting muscle and connective tissue.

- Lysine and Vitamin **C** together form L-carnitine, a biochemical mechanism that enables muscle tissue to use oxygen more efficiently therefore delaying fatigue.

- Aids bone growth by helping to form collagen (*the fibrous protein that makes up bone*) cartilage and other connective tissue.

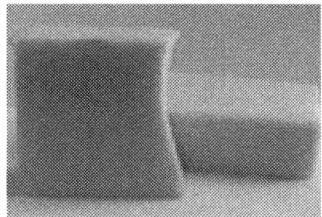

Cheese is a good source of protein

METHIONINE

- Precursor of cystine and creatine

- May increase antioxidant levels (*glutathione*) and reduce blood cholesterol levels.

- Helps remove toxic waste from the liver and assists in the regeneration of liver and kidney tissue.

PHENYLALANINE

- The major precursor of tyrosine.

- Enhances learning, memory, mood and alertness.

- Used in the treatment of some types of depression.

- It is a major element in the production of collagen

- Suppresses appetite.

THREONINE

- Helps detoxify dangerous substances

- Helps prevent fat build up in the liver

- Important component of collagen

- Generally low in vegetarians

CONDITIONALLY DISPENSABLE

They are conditionally dispensable based on the body's ability to actually synthesize them from other amino acids.

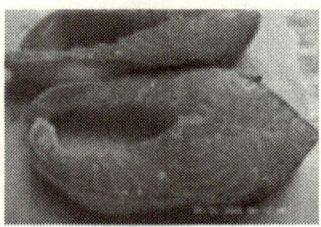

Salmons provides a good source of protein

ARGININE

- Can increase the secretion of insulin, glucagon, and growth hormones.

- Aids injury rehabilitation, formation of collagen and stimulates the immune system

- Precursor of creatine, gamma amino butyric acid **GABA** *(a neurotransmitter in the brain).*

- May increase sperm count and Y-lymphocyte response.

CYSTENINE

- Detoxifies harmful chemicals in combination with L-aspartic acid and L-citrulline.

- Helps prevent damage from alcohol and tobacco use.

- Stimulates white blood cell activity.

TYROSINE

- Precursor of the neurotransmitters dopamine, norepinephrine and epinephrine, as well as thyroid, growth hormones and melanin *(the pigment responsible for skin and hair color).*

- May help increase growth hormone secretion in high doses

- Elevates mood.

CYSTINE

- Contributes to strong connective tissue antioxidant actions

- Aids healing processes, stimulates white blood cell activity and helps diminish the pain from inflammation

- Essential for the formation of skin and hair

GLUTAMINE
(*Most abundant amino acid*)

- Plays a key role in immune system functioning

- An important source of energy, especially for the kidneys and intestines during caloric restriction

- May act as a neurotransmitter in some areas of the brain and retina

- Powers the brain, aids memory, stimulates intelligence and sustains concentration

HISTIDINE

- One of the major ultraviolet-absorbing compounds in the skin

- Important in the production of red and white blood cells; used in the treatment of anaemia

- Used in the treatment of allergic diseases, rheumatoid arthritis and digestive ulcers.

PROLINE

- A major component in the formation of connective tissue and heart muscle

- Readily mobilized for muscular energy

- Major constituent of collagen

DISPENSABLE AMINO ACIDS

Dispensable amino acids, also called non-essential amino acids, can be synthesized by the body from other amino acids namely: -

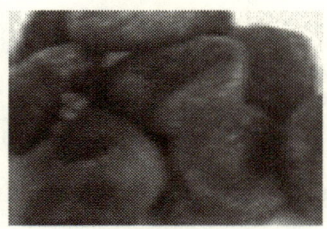

Dried figs are good sources of plant protein

ALANINE

- Fortifies the major component of the connective tissue

- Very active in the glucose-alanine cycle, which allows muscles and other tissues to derive energy from amino acids

- Promotes healing

- Helps strengthen up the immune system.

ASPARAGINE

- Ensures the body's ability to maintain good health and vitality

- Helps the nervous system to sustain equilibrium

- Important in the metabolism of ammonia

- Important in the biosynthesis of glycoprotein

ASPARTIC ACID

- Helps convert carbohydrate into muscle energy

- Aids in immune system and liver function

- Builds the immune system, immunoglobulin and antibodies

- Reduces ammonia levels after exercise.

GLYCINE

- Aids in the manufacture of other amino acids and is part of the structure of haemoglobin and cytochromes *(enzymes involved in energy production)*

- Has a calming effect and is sometimes used to treat manic-depressive and aggressive individuals

- Produces glucagon, which mobilizes glycogen

- Can inhibit sugar cravings

GLUTAMIC ACID

- A major precursor of glutamine, proline, ornithine, arginine, glutathione and GABA

- A potential source of energy

- Aids in the absorption and elimination of fats

- Important in brain metabolism and metabolism of other amino acids

SERINE

- Important in the production energy within the cells

- Aids memory and nervous system function

- Helps build up immune system by producing immuno-globulins and antibodies

FORM AND FUNCTION OF PROTEIN AND AMINO ACIDS

NATURE, SIGNIFICANCE AND NEED

Free - Form

Helps prevent muscle catabolism, requires no digestion, easily and quickly absorbed into the blood stream which makes it readily available for performing athletes.

Hydrolyzed - Long chain

This is well broken down or predigested - long chain amino acids, and in this form aids the rapid entry into the digestive system, examples of this are whey and lactalbumin.

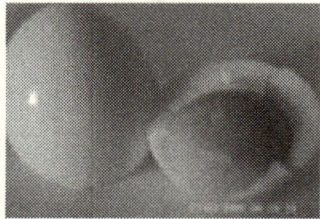

Eggs provides a rich source of protein

Branched -Chain

During training, branch chains assist in the formation of alanine from glucose, which in turn helps prevent catabolism or atrophy normally associated with inadequate glucose in the system.

Di - and Tripeptides

Di-Tripeptides are very important to athletes because they have the ability to increase the level of nitrogen retention in the body. These are two to three molecule amino acids that are rapidly digested depending on the its derivative and availability

Plant foods

Natural source of protein from seeds, nuts, fruits, vegetables and tubers, often with Fibre. Very low in certain essential aminos, for example Methionine, takes a long time to digest and for absorption to take place.

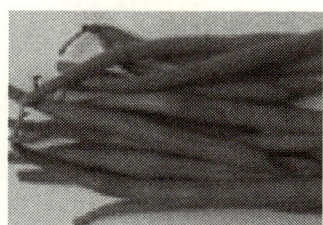

Green beans a good source of plant protein

Animal foods

Sources are from ruminants or herbivorous animals. Containing all essential amino Acids! Readily digested but absorption takes longer, especially with fatty meats.

BETTER UNDERSTANDING OF AMINO ACIDS

Despite so many varieties of amino acid products in the form of food supplements, currently available to athletes requiring additional protein. (And not anabolic-androgenic steroids) Most if not all, still find buying the right amino acids to be quite confusing and difficult.

Here are some basic facts that can help a lot of serious minded athletes work through the confusion.

Types of free – form amino acids (available commercially)

1) **Pure crystalline amino**

   This supplement offers the highest biological value within the system and should at all times be the athlete's first choice. It is more effective in achieving specific results from individual or isolated aminos, however is usually more expensive

2) **Peptide –Bonded aminos**

   These are classified as multiple aminos and very essential when it comes to improving the efficiency ratio of dietary protein.

Note: **Do not purchase these products if your expectation is to gain maximum effects from individual or isolated amino acids.**

- Protein powders and mixed amino acids will usually enhance an athlete's basic dietary protein intake. They are used primarily by strengthen athletes – namely power lifters and bodybuilders who want to develop greater musculature or maximise strength.

- Powder, blended in a drink offers an easy- to - absorb balanced mixture of all the amino acids that make up complete protein. Use these products with a complementary vitamin, co- factors and co-enzymes for increased effectiveness.

- Use individual amino acids to achieve specific effects. Start with small dosages and increase levels gradually. Do not exceed the recommended dose.

- Try to use products designed scientifically with the athlete in mind. Inexpensive supplements often mean lower quality for example, *"incomplete proteins"*.

- Look for pure, hypo – allergenic supplements, and products that contain no chemical additives, artificial colours or sweeteners.

- Be sure to supplement with vitamin B6 whenever you take amino acids. This vitamin is an essential co-factor necessary for the metabolism of protein.

NOTE: As a matter of fact there is however no reasonable damage to the health of an athlete who consumes a considerable amount of protein. Remember that the Estokimos thrive on a diet in which protein predominates. Again, there is no evidence or proof whatsoever that a high protein diet predisposes them to cancer or other organic diseases. Again, in the days of the cave man and later during his nomadic existence, his diet was largely protein. However, cancer is on the increase today even with less protein consumption, as compared with the earlier times in man's history.

Chapter Two
CARBOHYDRATE FOR ATHLETE ON A MISSION!

You have chosen to work hard with the aim of becoming successful in the world of sport and to achieve your objectives without the use/misuse/abuse of any anabolic-androgenic or stimulating substances that are best known to pharmacists.

As a serious minded athlete on a mission, it is time to propel your training and nutritional programme towards maximum performance and to do it correctly, safely and through natural sources you have to start with the right nutritional fuel and that fuel is *carbohydrate.*

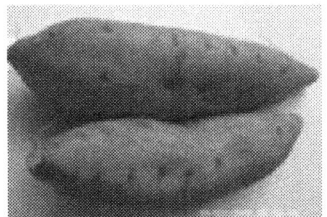

Sweet potatoes are a good source of carbohydrate

Research recognises carbohydrate, as one of the human body's most energy generating substances, which attempts to balance *"the energy in with the energy out"*. The former refers to the amount of carbohydrate ingested, the later refers to how many calories from carbohydrate you expend due to metabolism, training and day-to-day activities. Also, success in sport depends on having an advantage over your fellow competitors by always being able to draw upon an added energy reserve that should come from *"MAJOR SOURCES"* of carbohydrate when you need it most This is essential – especially during intense training and competition.

- Glycogenesis - is the conversion of glucose to glycogen when the glucose in the blood exceeds demand. Glycogen is one form in which the body fuel is stored for later use usually in the muscle tissue or the liver.

- Gluconeogenesis - is the formation or the process of synthesizing of glucose from amino acids and triglycerides.

Again, considerable research has shown that carbohydrate acts as spark plug for your body's restorative and recuperative powers. This is all the more reason why an athlete must consume sufficient energy yielding carbohydrates that can provide the fuel needed for-:

- Vital explosive power, prolonged endurance, increased stamina, energy and strength

- Decrease the time needed to recover from a rigorous training regimen

The brain, central nervous system and other tissues rely heavily on a constant supply of carbohydrate to satisfy the immediate and long- term energy demands imposed on them.

THE PERFORMANCE POWERHOUSE

Training long hard hours without a high energy level and sufficient fuel from carbohydrate, will surely disrupt your determination to go beyond and to reach the height that you have set for yourself. At this point, you have to bear in mind that your muscle uses glucose during training and competition and is essential and critical for two of the most desired results in sport-:

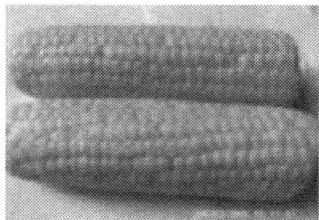

Maize a good source of glucose (Monosaccharide)

- Performance - energy production for muscular work

- Anabolic processes within muscle cells

At any point in time, if sufficient carbohydrate is not in the system, then the body will have no choice than to consume protein for energy production. Remember that protein is supposed to -:

- Build muscle tissue

- Build and rebuild worn out tissues

Inadequate consumption of carbohydrate therefore will surely result in a self defeating act.

Our researchers believe that the best way to replenish carbohydrate is to eat a high carbohydrate meal. This kind of meal is the best choice especially when an athlete intends to maintain a vital and rich carbohydrate stores in his muscles and liver. A high performance diet in an athlete's meal should contain up to 45 – 65% carbohydrate.

Note: A slice of whole wheat bread weighing 31.25grams contains approximately 13 grams of carbohydrates equal to about 52 calories (calories per gram = 4*) so (13 x 4 = 52).

Every serious minded athlete should note that glucose should be the most important nutrient to focus on before, during and after training. For example, if you eat refined and processed carbohydrate *(like white bread and most packaged carbohydrate foods)* this can lead to a lack of sustainable nutrients in your diet that are needed to pay the price for the heavy duty training regimen you put yourself through.

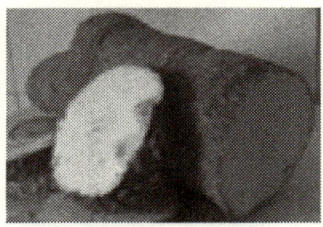

Yam provides an excellence source of carbohydrate (Starch)

Any athlete training to make an impact in the world of sport, must bear in mind that if he consumes too little carbohydrate at any point under any intense training programme, will result in glycogen stores being depleted and the body then enters a detrimental state. This will result in amino acids from protein being used to make glucose. Again, this is dangerous and should be avoided because eating too little carbohydrate wastes protein, distorts the growth and development associated with a good training regimen which is needed for optimum performance in order to win championships.

A sound and viable body has 1, 500 – 3,000 stored calories of carbohydrates in the form of muscle and liver glycogen and over 100,000 stored calories in body fat. However, taking insufficient carbohydrate especially during training will deliberately place your muscle gain, metabolism and energy at risk not to mention some potentially negative *ketogenic* – related activities.

MAJOR SOURCES OF CARBOHYDRATES

Monosaccharide:

These remain the simplest form of all carbohydrates, or sugars. They are essential nutrients for your recovery and are easily absorbed into the body, also assist in the process of - regenerative production of Adenosine Triphophate *(A.T.P).*

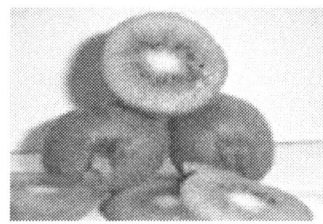

Kiwi fruit are a good source of (Monosaccharide)

(i) Glucose (or Dextrose)

Carbohydrate, the body's preferred fuel source must be changed or digested into glucose before it can be of use to the body. Glucose as it is usually referred to, can be found naturally in food and in most if not all carbohydrate origins.

(ii) Fructose (or levulose):

The sweetest form of the simple sugar is fructose also called fruit sugar and appears in large amounts in fruits and honey.

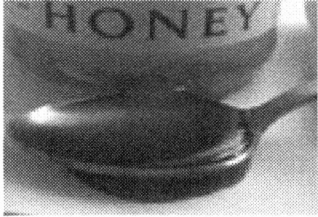

Honey a very rich fruit sugar (Monosaccharide)

(iii) Galactose

This simple-sugar is not likely to be found in a natural free - form. Conversely, galactose binds with glucose to form milk sugar or lactose.

Disaccharide:

Disaccharide or "double sugar" cannot be utilised by the body as such, it must be changed or digested. In most cases two monosaccharide are united chemically, at least one of which is glucose and forms these simple sugars.

(i) Sucrose (table sugar):

It is the most common of the simple sugars, and is present in naturally occurring carbohydrate foods like honey, cane sugar, beets and maple syrup. It is a combination of glucose and fructose to form sucrose.

(ii) Lactose (Milk sugar):

The least sweet of the simple sugars and occurs naturally in milk. The digestive problems or the intolerance of lactose is a result of insufficient quantities of an enzyme called lactase which is responsible for splitting galactose and glucose.

(iii) Maltose (Malt sugar):

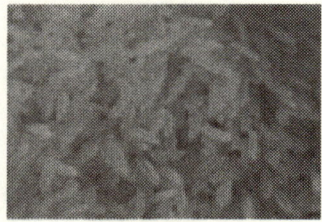

Rice provides good source of maltose (Disaccharide)

This is the combination of two glucose (or Dextrose) molecules to form "maltose" or malt sugar. The digestion or fermentation of starch *(another form of carbohydrate)* in the alimentary canal can also produce maltose, other sources include: cereals, germinating seeds and malt liquors alternatively referred to as beer.

MILK AND LACTOSE INTOLERANCE

"Milk is fattening, hard to digest, a risk for heart damage and is only for kids". Most of this advice has prevented athletes from consuming milk which is so needed for their overall health and vitality. This kind of thinking and campaigning has given milk a poor image. Milk in any

capacity remains a life sustaining food, rich in calcium – protein, vitamin A, D and B12.

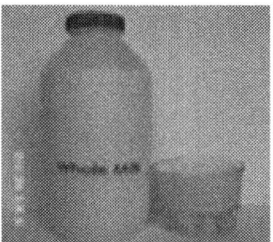

Milk is a good source of lactose (Disaccharide)

New studies show that the calcium in milk may help lower cholesterol, controls hypertension, prevents heart attacks and certain cancers. Its other properties are to strengthen bones, cartilage and collagen. Despite these obvious scientifically proven facts, many athletes still believe that milk interferes with their training; also that milk and certain milk products will make them develop gas and diarrhoea.

This is due to the lack of an enzyme called "Lactase", which is needed to digest milk sugar. As a result of this, many athletes are unable to enjoy the benefits that accompany milk and other dairy products.

In the interest of health, vitality and longevity associated with performance, you need to start drinking milk. All athletes at every level need calcium *(not to mention the proteins and vitamins)*. The amount of fat in milk and milk products depends on the type you consume. The fat in whole milk is actually fattening, but low fat or non-fat products can be a boost to the building of muscle tissue.

Milk is an excellent source of high quality protein that supplies essential amino acids. Milk contains the B vitamin riboflavin that helps convert food into energy and any intense training program requires an abundance of it. Milk has calcium, along with the necessary vitamins- A, B, D and phosphorous, to build and maintain a strong skeletal structure.

Note: A calcium supplement is not at any level or capacity comparative to milk.

Whole milk contains about 3% fat by weight, 53% of total calories compared to 1 – 2% for low – fat milk and for non fat milk. Cheese and yoghurt made from whole milk contains a high percentage of fat, whereas those from skimmed milk contain very little fat. A glass of low fat milk has only 100 calories, which makes it easy to fit several glasses into any diet program.

Finally, a glass of whole milk contains about 25 milligrams of cholesterol, one – tenth of that can be found in an egg. Non fat milk, having no fat to carry the cholesterol - therefore has no cholesterol.

POLYSACCARIDES:

Also known as complex carbohydrate, these are a result of many or multiple simple sugars chemically linked together. Endurance athletes, such as marathon runners, road runners, long distance cyclists and other athletes that are involved in gruelling training schedules require easily digestible food whist performing progressively. As a matter of fact, make sure that your energy sources are from low glycemic index carbohydrates.

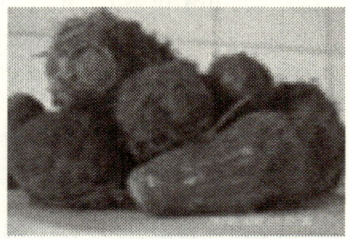

Cocoyam provides a good source of starch (Polysaccharide)

These complex bonds make them ideal for prolonged energy demands, such as during a workout, due to their slow digestive process and the muscle's requirement for carbohydrate. They remain a durable primary fuel source. So my fellow athletes throw away those ephedrine pills and start taking simple and complex carbohydrates that will help promote an immediate and sustained energy release.

(i) Starch:

This complex carbohydrate is present in all cereals, peas, beans, potatoes and so on. When therefore, you eat a plant food, your body system will automatically break it down into a usable energy source which can be utilised to fuel varied training regimens.

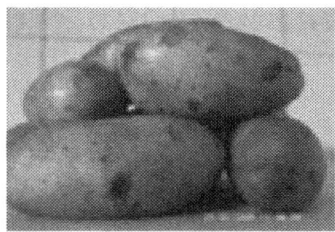

Irish potatoes are a good source of starch (Polysaccharide)

Again, some common examples of food containing large quantities of *starch* are as follows: grains, wheat and rice, *legumes* such as peas and beans, and *tubers* such as potatoes.

Note: Human beings actually store glucose as glycogen in the muscle, to be used as energy, whereas many plants store theirs as starch also for the same purpose.

"Dextrins" are formed from starch containing foods, as a result of exposure to strong dry heat, or the action of some digestive ferment. We find dextrin in the crusts of bread and in certain breakfast foods.

(ii) Fibre:

An efficient digestive system allows for the absorption of nutrients in your body to be smooth, quick and more efficacious. It also helps athletes benefit immensely from their nutritional intake and in so doing increases performance.

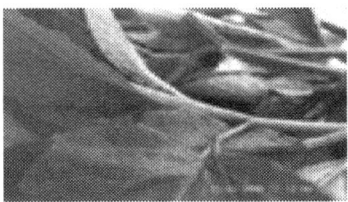

Green leafy vegetables are excellent sources of insoluble fibre

High fibre diets have been linked to a lower incidence of obesity. These complex carbohydrates exist only in plants and are a crucial component in digestion and health.

FIBRE AND DIGESTION

Incidentally, it is nature and not human beings that invented fibre. Brothers and sisters in sport, are you getting enough from your diet? Sportsmen should endeavour to consume at least 20 – 35grams of fibre per day. Also to capitalise on these benefits – athletes will need both

- Soluble - *for the blood sugar effect*

- Insoluble - *for smooth gastrointestinal absorption*

Soluble fibres help control blood sugar levels in the system while insoluble help regulate the digestive process and at the same time bind with fats, making them less absorbed.

Once more, insoluble fibre is a solid defender against colon cancer, dilutes colonic contents so that carcinogen substances loose some potency and improves the body's ability to control blood sugar levels by positively regulating the digestion and absorption of carbohydrate.

- *Soluble fibres include pectins, gums and oat bran.*

- *Insoluble fibres include wheat bran roughage and vegetable cellulose.*

Note: "If you are eating a large amount of protein and fat, fibre can easily become neglected"

It should be noted that cruciferous vegetables like cauliflower, broccoli and brussels sprouts are all low fat, high in fibre that actually improves the digestion of everything else you eat. Make sure you include: fresh fruit, beans and wheat-based products as well, since they are an excellent source of fibre to ensure a healthy digestive system.

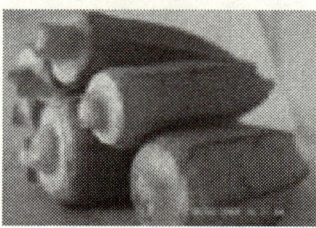

African okro is a good source of insoluble fibre

(ii) Glycogen.

This consists of large number of blood sugar molecules linked together and is fundamentally a polysaccharide of animal origin, stored in the muscle as glycogen. The other important storage depot is the liver; glycogen is also referred to as complex carbohydrate.

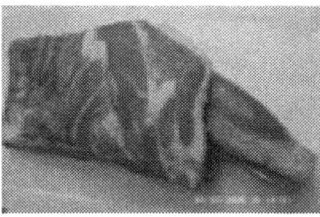

Lean meat is an excellent source of glycogen (Complex carbohydrate)

The build up of muscle glycogen can sustain high levels of energy for several hours and is very important during prolonged high intensity training resulting in a high competitive level of performance. Muscle glycogen is ideal for all sportsmen and women who require a safe and natural increase in oxygen carrying capacity. Sufficient glycogen in the muscle will surely and steadily help to provide the required advantage by increasing the level of Adenosine Triphospahte (ATP). This is a high energy compound that powers muscle contraction during concentric and eccentric workouts.

Athletes at all levels can sustain exertion, increase work, dynamically reduce fatigue, improve endurance and strength when adequate glycogen is taken at regular intervals.

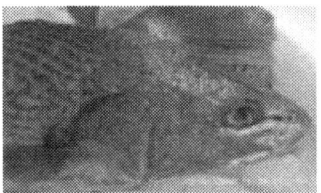

Lean fish provides good sources of glycogen (Complex carbohydrate)

Note: Safe and natural glycogen is excellent for preventing protein and muscle tissue from being used for energy and is a key element in energy production.

Whenever you feel weakness in your muscles it is because your muscle glycogen stores or blood sugar levels are low. We have observed that muscle glycogen levels become progressively lower as a result of intense training.

As glycogen levels decrease, the athlete's energy depleted, causing muscle soreness, premature fatigue, halting training intensity and enthusiasm.

Most coaches have failed to realise that the first two hours of recovery after intense exercise actually proves to be the most crucial time in the replacement of depleted fuel stores. During this period, the body is most capable of storing glycogen for later use. More so, if the body experiences weakness and fatigability before the next training programme; in other words runs out of fuel. I can personally assure you that it is going to be the *"sustain released"* complex carbohydrate that is lacking.

At this stage it should be known by all athletes that what goes into the body before and after their training is critical and it is the difference between a champion and a champion to be.

Chapter Three
FAT – THE NATURAL ENERGY DEPOT

Make no mistake about it, we all need fat in our diet and we cannot survive or become a champion without them. Fat provides insulation and energy and protects important body organs. Serves as a solvent for the transport of fat soluble vitamins and is an essential supplier of fatty acids. Without fat, the body cannot synthesise certain crucial hormones, such as testosterone and at the same time maintain the structure of the muscle and skeletal cells. As you can see, fat issue is so essential to our overall well-being.

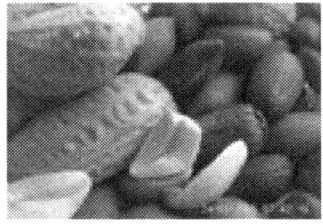

Peanuts are a good sources of phospholipids (Unsaturated fatty acids)

All fats have glycerine as part of their molecular structure. Fat are composed of glycerine and acids, called fatty acids. There may be one, two or more fatty acids combined chemically with glycerine to form fat. Some samples of fatty acids are:

- Oleic acid in olive oil

- Butyric acid in butter

- Caprylic acid in vegetable margarine

- Palmitic and Steric acids in mutton fat.

Also, note that the fat of various animals and plant foods are different because of the nature of the fatty acids present in them.

MORE FUEL MORE ENERGY

Dietary fat is either saturated, monounsaturated or polyunsaturated. These words confuse athletes, coaches and some sport administrators. As a result, almost all the total calories of fats consumed by our athletes are saturated, whereas the greatest percentage of fat intake should be polyunsaturated.

A complete meal needs a precise amount of fat for energy, metabolism and health. In the same vein, do not starve yourself of fat because the correct amount of appropriate fats is essential for optimum performance. Fat also contributes to feelings of satiety and pleasure during eating in variety of diets.

As an example: 0.48 grams per pound of bodyweight*, or about 18% -23% of total calories is ideal for a champion to be at all levels.

Note*: **Numerous clinical studies have shown that when higher amounts of good fats, such as essential Fatty Acids (EFAS) are included in your diet, your metabolism increases and as does your protein synthesis.**

Adequate fat will increase energy production but chronically consuming too much fat has also been linked to several metabolic and life – threatening diseases, such as diabetes, cerebrovascular and cardiovascular disease. The prevalence of some cancers is also said to have a considerable link with a diet high in fat. Consuming too little fat however, can also cause problems such as: abnormal testosterone production and symptoms of fat- soluble vitamin malnutrition (A, D, E and K) can arise.

Note: **One large slice of bacon contains approximately 5 grams of fat.**

Calories per gram = 9*

(5 x 9 = 45)

Equal to 45 calories from fat

MAJOR SOURCES OF FAT

Triglyceride – is the major source of dietary fat *(saturated, polyunsaturated and monounsaturated fats)* and is usually stored in adipose tissue. Triglycerides are either used for energy or stored as body fat. Fortunately, excess calories, no matter what form they take, can be easily converted by your liver to triglycerides.

Triglycerides are typically divided into two types for the sake of clarification.

a) Glycerol:

It is an alcohol that may not constitute a fat because of its solubility in water. Better still, glycerol assumes the characteristics of a carbohydrate, equating to approximately 4 calories per gram.

b) Fatty Acids:

Chemically, these are organic acids composed of carbon atoms with hydrogen molecules attached to them. The actual nature of fatty acids largely depends on the number of hydrogen molecules linked to them at any point in time. For example, the more hydrogen attachments, the more saturated the fat becomes - in other words more solid.

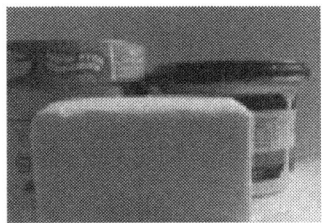

Butter is a good example of (Saturated fatty acids)

Note: There are essentially three 3 fatty acids that your body can not produce by itself and are:

- Arachidonic Acid

- Linoleic Acids

- Linolenic Acids

Types of Fatty acids.

(i) Saturated fatty acids:

The reason for the term *"saturated fatty acid"* is simply because it holds as many hydrogen atoms as is chemically possible. Unfortunately this is not a very good dietary composition for the athlete's performance. Many animal products such as beef, lamb and pork contain a high percentage of saturated fats, and indeed some vegetable sources are also high in saturated fats which are detrimental to the overall performance of a champion to be.

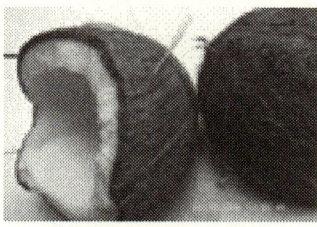

Coconut oil is a good example of (Saturated fatty acids)

Note: You can use butter, palm and coconut oil during training but not during competition, because these are extremely high in   saturated fats. Again, meat fats and butter are example of saturated fat that is usually solid at room temperature.

Unfortunately, too much body fat and a high intake of dietary fat are often linked to cancers of the uterus, ovaries, prostate, colon and breast.

(ii) Unsaturated fatty acids:

There are two reasons why this fatty acid is called unsaturated

(a) Its holds less hydrogen atoms when compared to a saturated fatty acid.

(b) It is not totally saturated with hydrogen atoms.

These are a *"good" and "acceptable"* form of fat that makes the difference between a winner and loser in a championship, and should constitute the greatest percentage of the entire fat intake.

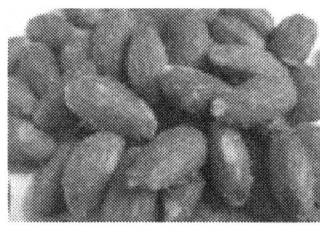

Almonds are a good source of (Monounsaturated fatty acid)

Examples*: - of monounsaturated fatty acid Olive oils canola oil, almonds and pecans.*

Examples: - *of polyunsaturated fatty acids or (omega – 3 and omega – 6 fatty acids) Soya, fish, sunflower and corn oil.*

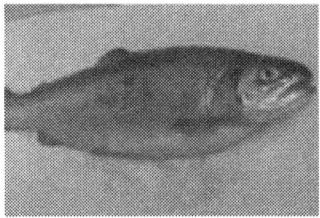

Fish of these kinds are a good source of (Polyunsaturated fatty acids)

Note: Unsaturated fats can be easily chemically manipulated and in so doing are potentially more harmful to your health than even saturated fats.

The ability of science to change the natural structure of food has never escaped consequence .However, it is wise and reasonable to note that changing the placement of hydrogen atoms *(as in partially hydrogenated fat or a trans- fatty acid)* can be detrimental to the overall interest of athletes especially in relation to their performance.

Phospholipids:

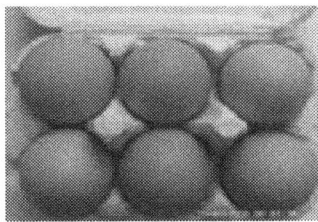

Eggs provide good sources of phospholipids (Unsaturated fatty acids)

These fats are extremely important to the health and vitality of sportsmen and women irrespective of which sport he/she may be involved in. These can be found in foods such as eggs, liver, soybeans, peanuts and wheat germ. Very important in maintaining the structural integrity of cells and plays a crucial role in blood clothing. They help to mobilise fatty acid distribution within the body and facilitate the utilisation of cholesterol.

Sterol:

Simple as it sounds though not so much of a known fatty acid within the sports circle, sterol remains a regulator of hormones in the body system and has many important functions such as:

- Hormonal balance

- Smooth metabolism

- Mood Regulator

- Neurotransmission in the brain.

Note: Cortisols come from sterols - vitamin D is also considered a sterol.

UNFORTUNATE FAT DICHOTOMY

Excess body fat is nothing more than the result of overeating or under training *(The more you eat the more you exercise, and the less you eat the less you exercise)* therefore increase your training, reduce your calories and you can only loose weight and not mass. In some circumstances, thyroid problems and hormonal imbalances can cause excess body fat to be stored. This can result in extreme fatigue and drowsiness when reducing calories.

Conceivably, when reducing calories it is vital to reduce your fat and carbohydrate intake and most importantly, is for you to increase your protein intake; otherwise you will end up burning up muscle tissue for energy. In addition to this, avoid all simple sugars, such as glucose, sucrose, and maltose if possible. Stick to complex carbohydrates like rice and potatoes. Also when cutting down on fat remember to include essential Fatty acids (EFAS)

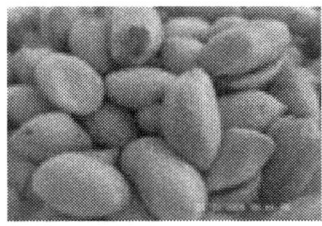

Groundnuts are good and essential source of (Monounsaturated fatty acid)

Warning: Avoiding simple sugar will prevent blood sugar fluctuation, which in turn reduces or prevents heavy insulin surges that cause easy fat storage.

On the one hand, lack of good or sufficient fat can provoke catabolism which in turn can cause muscle discomfort, shrinkage of muscle tissue and may even lead to injury. So, to keep the training intensity high, you must ensure that you strike a balance between too much and too little fat.

Note: The average 79.5kgs person stores about 110,740 calories (12.300g).

To enjoy a reasonable fat loss, two major processes must occur-:

(a) The mobilisation and circulation of stored fats in the body must increase.

(b) Fat must be transported and converted to energy at the powerhouse site of cell *"the mitochondria"*

In doing so, your stamina and energy will increase by the amount of fat that is broken down and transported to the muscle where it can be burned as fuel.

Chapter Four
VITAMINS – THE PROTECTIVE NUTRIENTS

Sports Scientists and nutritional experts are always researching the role of vitamins in relation to sports performance and the overall well being of the athletes. From every angle of understanding, they do actually encourage sportsmen and women to include in their diet a multivitamin or a vitamin tablet each day. However, they also emphasise that athletes do not need to swallow supplements upon supplements under any guise if they eat correctly.

Pills do not and will not provide the sort of energy you get from balanced and nutritious diet.

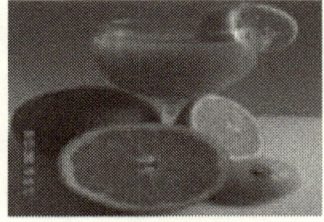

Pure orange juice from concentrates is rich in vitamins

Note: Taking multivitamins is important for a performing athlete, but not as substitute for food.

Vitamins are essential non – mineral substances in minute quantities helping the body system to maintain and sustain normal metabolic development. Without their existence, or if they are lacking as a result of insufficiency in our diet, then our growth and overall development will eventually be rendered useless. Vitamins differ chemically from one to another, especially in the way they aid the body's biomechanical system.

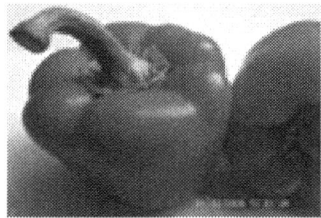

Peppers are rich in vitamins, example (Vitamin C, ascorbic acid)

Vitamins are also referred to as catalysts, and this is because of their ability to modify the velocity of both the chemical and physical processes in the body system. To always enjoy this wholesome package to its fullest, athletes should endeavour to derive their vitamins from natural food sources. It is important for athletes to understand that some vitamins are destroyed by heat, whilst others are not. Some are water soluble, whilst others are fat soluble.

Note: Vitamins are an insignificant energy source, that is to say very small or zero in calories. However they are needed to prevent diseases and infection and to keep performance on the right track, since insufficient will definitely put all gain and development associated with performance to an end.

VITAMINS AND FUNCTIONALITIES

Vitamin A:

Also called 'retinal' a term which is derived from the retina of the eye? This is simply because the vitamin makes up the chemical "rhodopsin" which enables and enhances the ability to focus in dim light. It is essential for vision (particularly at night); Vitamin A aids cell development, maintenance of the cornea, bone, tooth growth reproduction and immunological regulation.

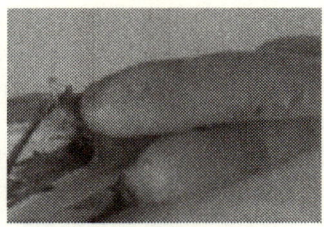

Carrots, a good source of vitamin A (Retinal)

Note: Vitamin A is soluble in fat and fat solvent (heat has no effect on this vitamin). Carotene is also converted into vitamin A, a change that takes place in the liver.

"Have you ever seen a rabbit with glasses"?

Eating a carrot a day may keep you away from the *opthamologist and cardiologist* or keep these specialists away from you! Note, it is the beta carotene of which carrots are a major source, that tends to reduce the risk of damage to the heart. The need for beta carotene depends on the kinds of activities we are engaged in. Excess is excreted, whilst large quantities are stored under the skin.

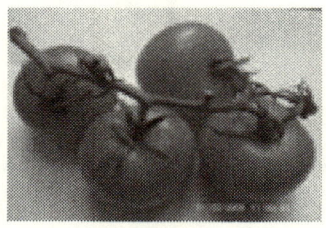

Tomatoes, an excellent source of vitamin A (Retinal)

Vitamin A and its pro - vitamins are found in:

Vegetables	*milk- whole*
Banana	*milk- evaporated*
Carrots	*oil, fish – body*
Tomatoes	*oil, fish – liver*
Apricots	*cheese*
Turnip green	*butter*
Egg yolk	
Liver	

If an athlete can keep in mind the foods in which Vitamin A is present in abundance, then it will be possible at all times to maintain a sufficiency of this important vitamin that is so essential for optimum health and vitality

IMPORTANCE OF VITAMIN B

The B vitamins are generally water soluble, responsible for the effective assimilation of protein, control stress and mood swings, keeps the skin healthy and maintains an even fluid balance. B complex formulas should contain all the other B vitamins in the correct ratio for optimum absorption and effect.

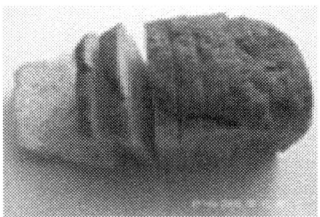

Bread is very rich in B vitamin

Note: Very high temperatures will surely destroy part or the entire B vitamin.

Also essential is vitamin B found in bread, but which is not destroyed by the process of baking.

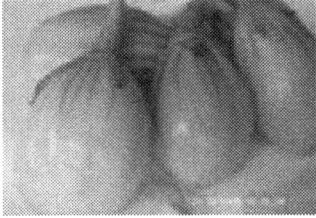

Garden eggs are rich in B vitamins and are good for the excretory system

Vitamin B or B vitamin, aids intramuscular and intravascular friction, enhances the nervous system, improves internal co-ordination between nerves and muscles. It also aids digestion, promotes growth, enhances muscular and energy production. *(Garden egg which is almost a neglected raw vegetable is among the range of vegetables which contains the highest quantity of Vitamin B.)*

VITAMIN B$_1$ THIAMINE:

This vitamin is water-soluble that must be replaced on a daily basis, as it is easily excreted. Found in skeletal muscle, enhanced with physical activity, the more you train the more it is used up.

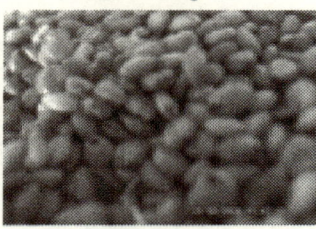

Guinea corn, a good source of vitamin B$_1$ (Thiamine)

Vitamin B$_1$ is needed to convert blood sugar into biological energy. It stimulates a metabolic reaction in the nerve tissue. Aids red blood cell formation and maintains the muscle tissues.

Available in the following:

Pork	*Millet*
Beef	*Guinea corn*
Liver	*Maize*
	Wheat

B$_1$ also requires other B complex vitamins in other to function efficiently and is especially beneficial in promoting a normal appetite and nervous system.

VITAMIN B$_2$ (RIBOFLAVIN):

Riboflavin is a co- enzyme that helps to energise the body and enable it to extract calories from fats, carbohydrates and proteins. It aids oxygen transfer to the tissues, and is crucial to energy production. It destroys toxins and detoxifies foreign organisms

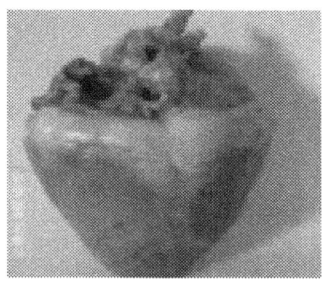

Glandular tissues like the heart are a good source of vitamin B$_2$ (Riboflavin)

Athletes, especially those undergoing vigorous training need riboflavin to help enhance the rapid production of red blood cells responsible for oxygen delivery (oxy-haemoglobin).

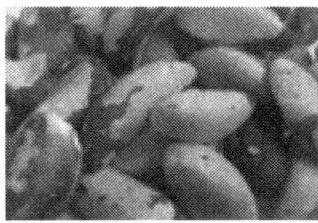

Brazil nuts provide a good source of vitamin B$_2$ (Riboflavin)

Important food sources are: glandular tissues also known as "Offal" (liver, heart, kidney, lungs etc)

Other good sources are -:

Eggs	milk
Cheese	yoghurt
Fish	meat
Whole grains.	

VITAMIN B$_3$ (NIACINAMIDE).

Niacinamide is a co – enzyme that enhances the delivery of oxygen to the body tissues and organs. Also aids a smooth, steady production and transportation of energy to the system.

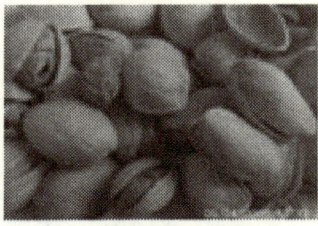

Pistachio nuts provide a good source of vitamin B$_3$ (Niacinamide)

Other important and crucial properties is its capability to directly increase the performance of any athlete that consumes enough of this vitamin.

Important sources are liver, kidneys and nuts of various origins contain this vitamin

VITAMIN B$_5$ (PANTHOTHENIC ACID):

Panthothenic acid is beneficial in recuperation, restoration and promotes the effective relaxation of an individual athlete involved in a strenuous day – to – day training regimen.

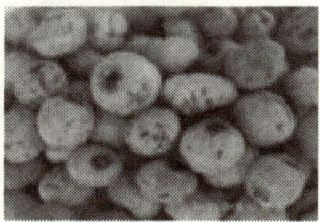

Tiger-nuts are good sources of vitamin B$_5$ (Panthothenic acid)

This vitamin is capable of metabolising carbohydrate and fat for energy production. It is usually called *(memory Vitamin)* because of its high concentration in the human brain. Best sources are: eggs, liver, kidney and other glandular tissue, whole grains, enriched breads and cereals, nuts.

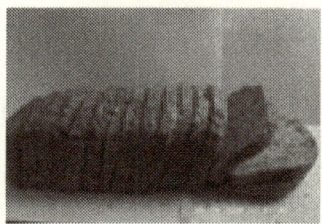

Enriched bread is a good source of vitamin B$_5$ (Panthothenic acid)

This vitamin is required to enhance the interaction between muscles, nerves and the overall physiological and anatomical functioning of the body system.

VITAMIN B₆ (PIRIDINE):

This co – enzyme is necessary for the conversion of muscle glycogen to glucose for energy production. B_6 metabolises proteins and amino acids in order to repair, build and rebuild new cells. It also helps to convert tryptophan to niacin which aids in the production of red blood cells. Important sources are whole grains:

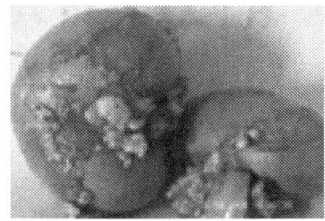

Glandular tissue like kidney provides a good source of B₆ (Piridine)

Cereals	*Kidney*
Millet	*Liver*
Guinea corn,	*Fish*
Maize	*Poultry*
Leafy green vegetables	*Shellfish*
Striated muscle	red meat

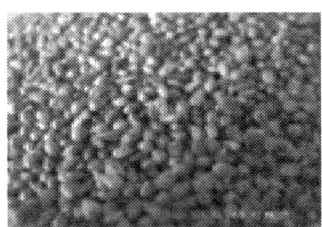

Millets is a good source of B₆ (Piridine)

Again, piridine is also referred to as *"the bodybuilding vitamin"* because of its intrinsic factor - that is its ability to stimulate proper utilisation of other important vitamins in the bodybuilding process. B_6 is responsible for the manufacture of hydrochloric acid (HCL) in the gut. Hcl is responsible for the breakdown and absorption of food in the body, but mainly that of protein.

Note: Athletes on a high protein diet should add B_6 in the form of B100 (supplementation). This would definitely make a difference in the absorption and utilisation of protein in the body.

VITAMIN B_{12} (CYANOCABALAMINE):

Its function is mainly as a co – factor in the process of digestion, synthesis, re-synthesis and effective absorption of nutrients into the body system, especially in the intestine. It also has intrinsic factors that are necessary for optimum growth and development required to sustain a healthy lifestyle.

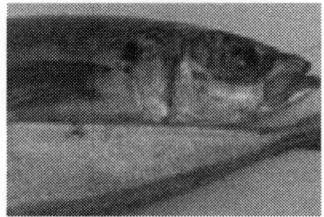

Fish of this type are a good source of B_{12} (Cyanocabalamine)

B_{12} (a co-enzyme) is critical in many key metabolic processes such as the synthesis of DNA and protein and most especially when training for strength, density and size.

Best sources are: *complete protein, e.g.: eggs, meat, fish, cheese, milk and shellfish*.

Other important functions of B_{12} are: the maintenance of nerve cells, assist in the breakdown of some fatty acids and is important for new cell synthesis.

BIOTIN:

This B complex vitamin helps to metabolise fat and carbohydrate for the energy needed for various physical activities that we involve ourselves in. It also breaks down some essential "amino acids" needed to build and rebuild muscle cells. Intense exercise usually places additional demands on Biotin.

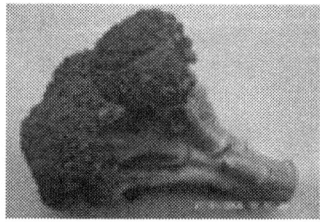

Broccoli provides a good source of biotin

Important food sources are as follows: brown rice, soyabeans and whole wheat bread. Biotin is generally distributed in foods.

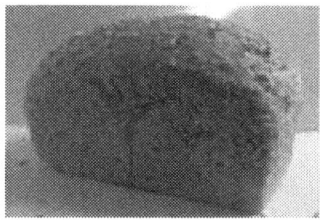

Whole wheat bread is a good source of biotin

B complex vitamins are required to enhance athletes in their workout by boosting energy output.

Examples: To promote *agility, stamina, endurance and for glycogen synthesis.*

FOLIC:

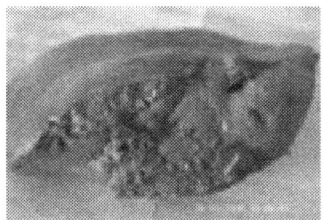

Glandular tissue like the liver, is very rich in folic acid

Partially aids red blood cell function, protects against cervical cancer and promotes new cell synthesis. Low levels of folic acid in the system may eventually result in a disease called *"Pernicious anaemia"*.

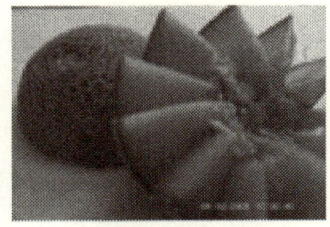

Water melon provides a good source of folic acid

Best food sources are: raw green leafy vegetables, raw fruits, seeds, legumes and liver.

VITAMIN C (ASCORBIC ACID):

An athlete deprived of this vitamin can develop swollen and sore gums, the teeth may become decayed. Deficiency can lead to joint pain, which may become very acute and almost unbearable on movement. Skin may develop bruising, patches and nose bleeds may occur. Vitamin C can prevent or cure all of these symptoms.

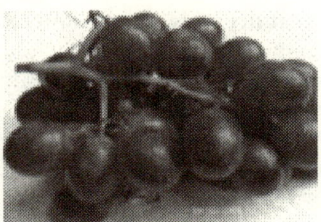

Grapes provide good sources of vitamin C (Ascorbic acid)

Vitamin C acts in two ways-:

- Firstly it functions as an anti-oxidant in the body and since free radicals can cause cell damage and stimulate the formation of cancer cells, low levels of vitamin C in the body allows for more oxidative damage to occur, thereby increasing the possibility of a normal cell mutating into a cancer cell

- Secondly, it can also protect the body from the effects of ageing and preserves the skin from infections.

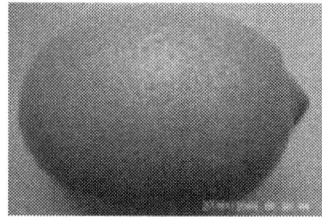

Lemon is a good source of vitamin C (Ascorbic acid)

Vitamin C performs the following function –:

- Promotes the absorption of iron

- Amino acid metabolism

- Thyroxin and collagen synthesis

Vitamin C plays a very important role in -:

- Decreasing blood cholesterol levels both directly and indirectly

- Preventing blood clots in the venous system

- Aids in the functioning of protein and helps in the prevention of cancer

- Helps to reduce cortisol and other stress hormones by lowering stress induced cortisol levels

Note: What is the greatest source of vitamin C?

Orange juice or other citrus fruits - (NO)

Answer: Vitamin C from "Tomato" is the best source.

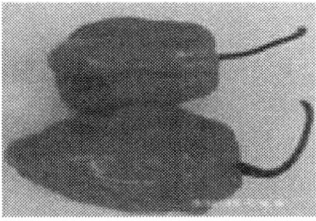

Peppers are good sources of vitamin C (Ascorbic acid)

Some important food sources are: the natural citrus varieties – oranges, tangerines, grapes, limes, lemons, cabbage, dark green vegetables, cantaloupe, berries, peppers, tomatoes and potatoes.

VITAMIN D (CALCIFEROL):

The sun does not have Vitamin D in its rays but the ultra violent rays therein convert precursors such as cholesterol, in the skin into active Vitamin D.

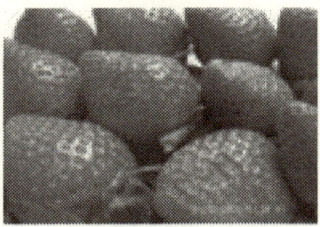

Berries provide a good source of vitamin D (Calciferol)

Note: Early morning self-synthesis with sunlight is reputed to be the best natural source of vitamin D.

Vitamin D usually called *"Sunshine Vitamin"* helps to regulate metabolism by-:

- Promoting the absorption of calcium and phosphate in the body system

- Helps to prevent osteoporosis *(weakness or loss of bone matrix)*

This vitamin is usually found in milk, cheese and other dairy products, performs especially in the mineralization of bone tissue, cartilage, tendons, ligament and other joint related tissue and cell formation.

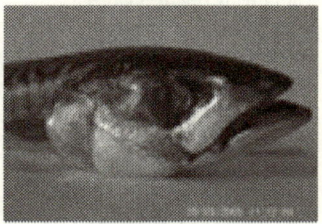

Oily fish is a good source of vitamin D (Calciferol)

Important food sources are fortified margarine, oily fish, eggs yolk, fortified milk and liver.

VITAMIN E (D ALPHA TOCOPHEROL):

This is a fat soluble vitamin and also a body lipid antioxidant. It prevents high levels of free radicals during intense exercise. It preserves and protects the skin from various forms of disease and infection. Also protects athletes against coronary heart disease and some types of cancer. Vitamin E is also capable of boosting the immune system.

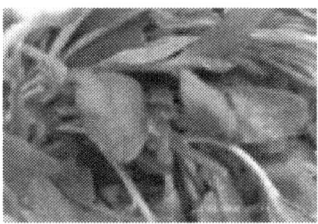

Water leaf vegetables are rich in vitamin A (Retinal)

Vitamin E is particularly helpful in the lungs, where cells receive maximal exposure to oxygen. This vitamin is also essential for muscle contraction and the stabilisation of cell membranes, also strengthens ligaments and tendons.

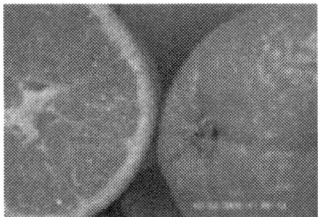

Oranges provides a good source of vitamin E (D alpha tocopherol)

Important food sources are as follows: leafy green vegetables, wheat germ, whole grains, liver, polyunsaturated plant oil, egg yokes, nuts, seeds, oranges and grapes.

VITAMIN K (MENADIONE):

Vitamin K helps in the synthesis of blood clotting proteins and proteins that regulate blood calcium *(thrombin and fibrin action in the mechanism of blood clotting).*

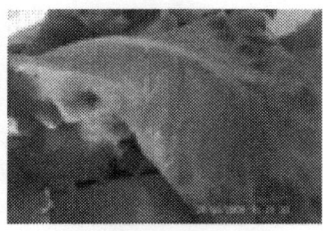

Cabbage provides a good source of vitamin K (Menadione)

This is another important fat soluble vitamin, which assists white blood cells to effectively prevent infection in the body. It is available in the intestine and helps to boost the action of free living micro – organisms therein.

Important food sources are: green natural cruciferous vegetables, raw fruits, cabbage, milk and liver.

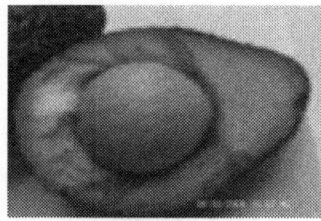

Raw fruits like avocados provide a good source of vitamin K (Menadione)

Chapter Five
ANATOMY OF MINERAL FUNCTIONALITIES

Minerals are micronutrients and absolutely essential for all hard training athletes who are interested in nothing but optimum performance, and are necessary for the body of sportsmen to function properly. For instance, muscle contraction, testosterone function, bone strength, oxygen transportation, maintenance of red blood cells count, efficient immunity and energy production, are all dependent on an adequate supply of minerals or micronutrients.

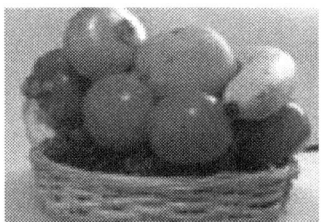

Fruits contain adequate minerals needed for healthy living

Note: High proportions of mineral, trace elements are rapidly lost during training and other strenuous day- to- day physical activities.

The incredible thing is that all too often researchers and doctors tend to ignore the significance and importance of minerals in the diet of an active sportsman. A lack of minerals can adversely affect the performance, regeneration of muscle growth, energy and vitality of the athletes in general.

Minerals act as antioxidants and are essential for hard training athletes. We all know that hard training of any kind results in the body producing free radicals, a kind of toxic waste resulting from the burning of energy and calories. When this waste is not eliminated, it can invariably cause damage to muscle cells and reduce recovery time.

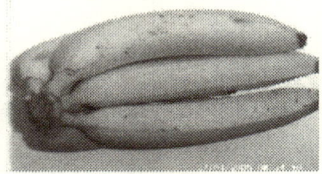

Banana is a good example of fruits rich in minerals

Furthermore, many athletes should know that over years their bodies build up heavy metals that are circulating and not absorbed into the system. This comes from lead from water pipes, aluminium pans, mercury fillings, and even from the air they breathe. This heavy metal build up causes premature fatigue, impairs sleep, lowers the immune system, causes memory loss, headaches and weakness of joints. To effectively remove and effortlessly excrete them requires a micronutrient element called a*" mineral"*.

UNDERSTANDING FUNCTIONS OF MINERALS

Below are some important facts that an athlete should know and more, about why the body should be provided with the finest micronutrient assistance possible. This will maximise the performance required to become a champion in any chosen field.

CALCIUM:

Constitutes 2% (by weight) of an adult body. Calcium absorption is between 10-30% under normal physiological conditions and most of that occurs in teeth and bones. Calcium also plays an important role in metabolism as a co-factor to Adenosine Triphosphate (ATP), and is instrumental in generating energy for the muscular and vascular contraction needed during training and competition.

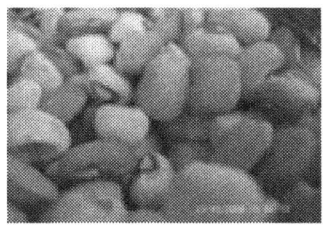

Beans provide good source of calcium

Calcium acts as an essential cofactor in various enzymatic conversions that occur during blood clothing. It is also essential for nerve transmission; maintaining fluid and electrolyte balance, supports cell integrity and improves the interaction between neurotransmitters.

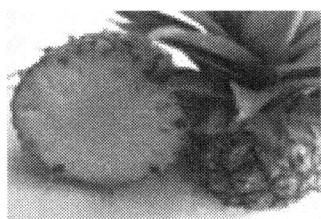

Pineapples and fruits in general provide a good source of calcium

Calcium is essential for bone strength and fortification, cartilage, collagen and maintaining strong teeth. Its directly reduces bone loss and preserves bone density. As a result of this, calcium is said to prevent half of all osteoporosis related hip fractures and severe osteoporosis applicable to the loss of bone density.

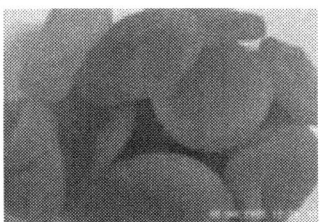

Soft dried apricots are a good source of calcium

Natural foods rich in calcium are:-

Vegetables, green	*egg yoke*
Peas	*malted milk*
Beans	*meats*
Legumes	*molasses*
Grains	*Fruits in general*
Gelatin	*Cheese*

SODIUM

Sodium is readily available in *"common salt"* or *"table salt"*, and is an essential element for athletes at any level whether competing or just simply to keep fit. Sodium is easily lost and must be reasonably replaced to avoid the malfunctioning of nerves and hormones. An athlete's diet must contain a reasonable amount at all times, the word *"reasonable*" is crucial as too much or too little can be of no benefit to vital organs like the heart, kidney and the liver.

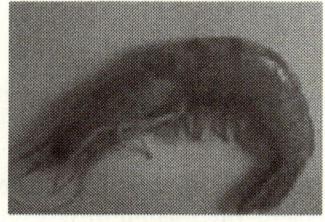

Oysters (Sea foods) are good sources of sodium

Note – Most foods in their natural state contain sodium and an athlete should not consume more than (4-5grams) equals 4000 – 5000mg per day.

1gram = 1000mg

4 gram = 4000mg

Mostly available in lot of natural food as follows:-

Sea foods	Lettuce
Broccoli	Oranges
Tomatoes	Nuts
Peanuts	Poultry
Butter	Vegetables
Cheese	Bananas
Pawpaw	Strawberries

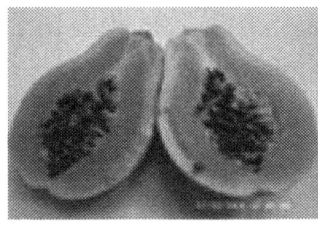

Natural raw fruits like pawpaw are rich in sodium

Sodium performs other functions as follows:

- Regulates fluid balance

- Promotes hormone efficiency

- Assist in nerve co-ordination

- Synergist muscle co-ordination

- Antagonist muscle inhibition

- Adrenaline, enzymatic and catalytic reactions

MAGNESIUM:

Magnesium is one of the most important and fourth most abundant mineral in the human body, exceeded only by sodium, potassium and calcium. Magnesium is an essential factor in the action of over 300 different enzymes in the body. That is why it is essential to the energy system. It has a direct effect on the nervous system, muscles and the heart.

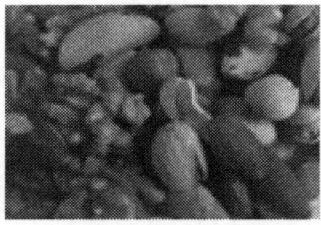

Nuts of various origins provide a good source of magnesium

Magnesium is important as a cofactor for enzymes that convert "ATP *to* ADP" *(Adenosine triphosphate to Adenosine diphosphate)* and also helps with the subsequent release and function of these enzymes. Magnesium is essential for reactions involving the synthesis and metabolism of carbohydrate, lipids, proteins and nucleic acids. A low level can cause many different effects

- Weakness and irritability are indications of its effects on the nervous systems

- Attention span and mental abilities may decrease

- Muscle twitching, tremors and a tendency for muscle cramps

- Loss of appetite, nausea and vomiting can result

- Severe depletion can cause cardiac arrhythmias

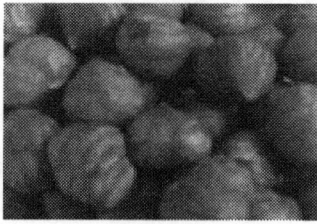

Hazelnuts a good source of magnesium

An athlete taking certain medication or abusing alcohol would be at risk of developing a magnesium deficiency.

Mostly available in many natural foods such as follows:-

Wheat bran	*Legumes*
Whole grains	*nuts*
Dark green vegetables	*cereals*
Dried fruit	*wheat germ*
Chocolate	*peas, dried*
Cocoa	*beans, dried*

PHOSPHOROUS:

Is a non-metallic element and is extremely important in human metabolism. Approximately 80% - 90% of phosphorous in the body combines to form calcium phosphate. This is used for the development of bones and teeth and is essential for energy transfer.

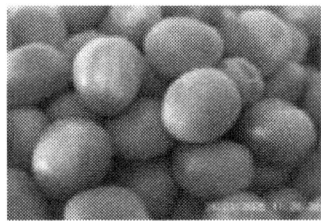

Peas are very rich in phosphorous

Phosphorous improves the body's ability to:-

- Deliver oxygen to contracting muscles

- Enhances the cardiovascular system's ability to deliver more nutrients to the muscles

Phosphorous is found in all cells of the body and is responsible for all parameters of life. It has a direct influence on growth, reproduction, absorption, respiration, excretion, muscle co-ordination and nerve conductivity.

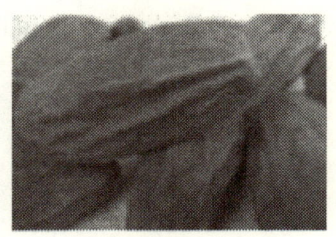

Dates nut are very rich in phosphorous

Phosphorous - best food sources of are:

Beans	*poultry*
Cereals	*Nuts*
Whole grain	*meats*
Pea's	*milk*
Dried Yeast,	*fish*
Wheat germ	*liver*
Chocolate, dark	*cheese*
Egg yolk	*gelatin*

POTASSIUM:

Potassium works in conjunction with other vitamins and minerals in order to carry out its essential function in the body system. This element maintains fluid and electrolyte balance, supports cell integrity, influences muscle contractions, promotes nerve impulse transmission and is a must for every serious minded athlete especially during training and competitions.

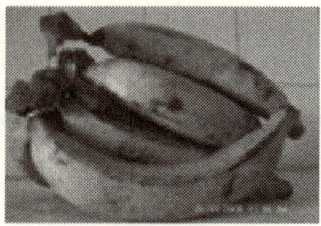

Plantain is rich in potassium

Every athlete should note that intense training and workouts place a direct demand on the body and increase the requirements of this crucial element.

Important natural sources are:

Meat	*melon*	*oranges*
Milk	*nuts*	*tangerines*
Honey	*beans*	*lettuce*
Banana		

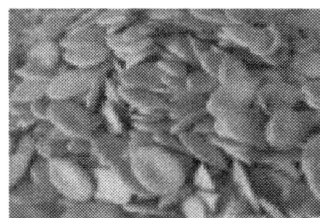

Melons provide a good source of potassium

Vegetables	*bananas*	*peas*
Grains	*limes*	*spinach*
Legumes	*grape*	*cocoa*
Fish	*olives*	*potatoes.*

ZINC:

Zinc functions similarly to potassium in many instances. However, the main function of zinc is to enhance and increase cell size of muscle tissue *(cell growth),* which is simply known as *"Hypertrophy".* Equally, insufficient levels of zinc in the body will adversely affect the strength of muscle tissue and will directly hinder performance at all levels of training and competition resulting in muscle shrinkage. This condition is referred to as *"Atrophy".*

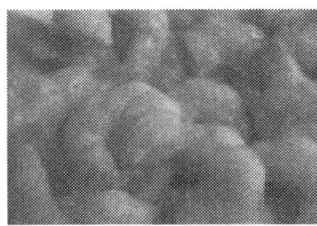

Shrimps are good source of zinc

Research shows that zinc is essential in the -:

- Making of *RNA and DNA*
- Crucial to the function of the immune system
- Transportation of vitamin A
- Promotes wound healing
- Involved in taste perception
- Enhances sperm and insulin production.

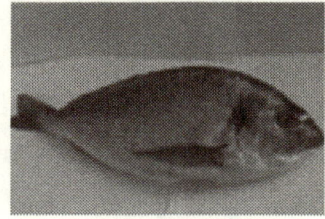

Fish are generally rich in zinc

Important food sources are: -

Eggs	*vegetables*
Oysters'	*whole grains*
Wheat	*Meats*
Fish	*Poultry*

IRON:

Women actually require less food than men, but not when it comes to winning championships. Recent research proves that sportsmen and women require equally protective foods, especially during moderate to high level training programmes.

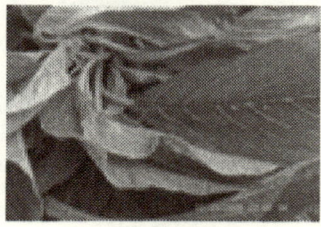

Leafy green vegetables provide excellent source of iron

Deficiency of iron in the body usually results to premature fatigue, sluggishness, dizziness and frequent fainting. Iron provides the major component of protein haemoglobin and myoglobin.

- Haemoglobin - oxygen transportation *(carries oxygen around your body)*

- Myoglobin - enhances muscle contraction. *(a protein in heart and skeletal muscles)*

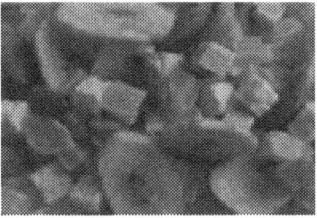

Dried fruits are rich in iron

Note: Lead elements and contamination especially from water can hinder the bioavailability of iron, which will reduce the haemoglobin carrying oxygen potential.

Important food sources are:

Red meat	*almond*	*green vegetable*
Fish	*liver*	*dried fruits*
Poultry	*heart*	*peas*
Shellfish	*kidney*	*coconuts*
Eggs	*Canned sardines'*	*oatmeal*

Chromium:

Main function is to activate insulin which is a powerful anabolic hormone and a chief promoter of energy and vigour. Chromium is called a *"stimulator"* because of it ability to mobilise the system during an intense training programme, that is to say chromium aids release of energy from glucose.

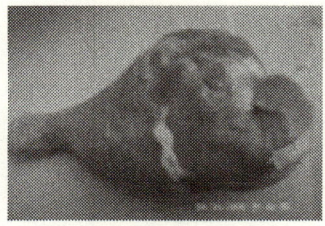

Turkeys are a good source of chromium

Food sources are:

Meats

Poultry

Animal and plant Fats

Vegetable oil of various origins

Turkey.

Natural foods

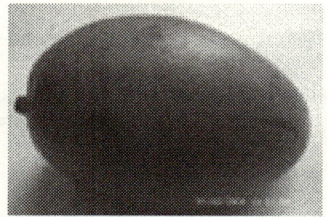

Fresh natural fruit like mangos are very rich in chromium

SELENIUM:

This element once in the body has the ability to penetrate muscular tissue and prevent damage caused by oxidation after intense exercise on a day – to – day basis. Selenium is a body preservative and age retardant element. It plays an important role in its ability to preserve the body's physiological and anatomical processes, prevents body malfunctions and acts as an anti – oxidant agent.

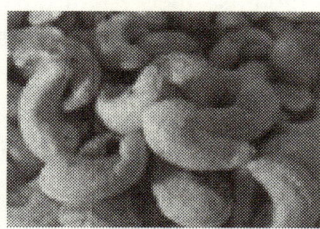

Cashew nuts are very rich in selenium

Also of importance is its ability to work in harmony with vitamin E.

Important food sources are

Shellfish

Oysters

Meat

Grains

Nuts

MOLYBDENIUM:

This mineral is crucial and bioavailable in many natural and unrefined foods, deficiency is unlikely and can be widely seen in many foods containing artificial colouring, flavouring, preservatives and chemical sweeteners.

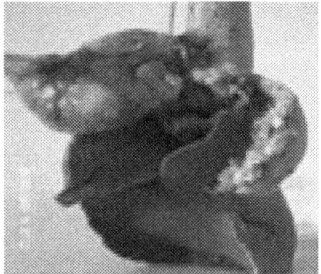

Glandular tissue such as the lungs are rich in molybdenum

Important natural food sources are: Legumes organ meat (offal) – liver, heart, kidney, lungs and cereals.

IODINE:

Iodine is another important mineral element because of its active role in the function of the thyroid gland. Its main function in the body is to effectively regulate growth, development and metabolism.

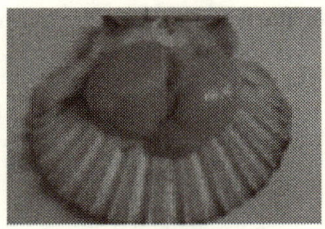

Sea foods (Salt fish) are very rich in iodine

Important food sources are: - iodise salt, seafood such as *Shellfish*, *Oysters*, bread and dairy products

Note: Because of its role in the functioning of the thyroid gland, inadequate levels result in goitre (swelling or mass on the throat).

Another physiological symptom includes – lethargy which for obvious reasons no athlete wants to experience.

Chapter Six
WATER – DRINK (H2O) YOU MUST!

The feeling of thirst is not a very good indication of how to effectively judge the body's hydration level. If you only drink water when you are thirsty, you are more likely to be a little or severely dehydrated.

This will reduce your energy output level and inhibit fat metabolism, which provides and sustains so much of the endurance and stamina you need during training and championships. Whilst water is critical to fat metabolism, protein digestion and oxygen function, too much water can dilute the concentration of digestive enzymes and acids and directly interfere with the process of nutrient digestion and absorption.

Note: The brain may misinterpret dehydration as lack of food, thereby stimulating appetite as a result.

Water is added to the body by drinking, in eating moist foods, by oxidising or the metabolising of protein, fats and carbohydrates. At the same time, water is lost from the body by visible and invisible perspiration from the skin during various physical activities, through urine and through faeces.

Competing athletes need a greater amount of water than an average individual. The reasons are as follows:

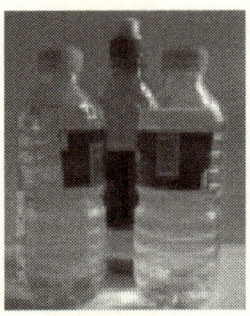

Clean water is a must for all

- *Water regulates and prevents dehydration.*

- *Adequate water is important for many metabolic and biochemical functions*

- *Assists in the formation of glycogen and the stimulation of protein synthesis.*

- *Helps the body to maintain normal cell volumes that are critical to sustaining muscle protein levels*

- *Keeps nervous membranes in the nose moist and helps to filter particles and air borne viruses that cause upper respiratory infections.*

They are two obvious and important facts, if an athlete intends to achieve the expected result at any stage of his career.

a) Firstly he must maintain hydration.

b) Secondly he must also drink clean water *(although not always abundant in some parts of the world).*

Note: Individuals can survive for weeks without food. But without water they will die in days. Also of importance to note is that 66% - 76% of your muscle weight is water, bones constitute 25% water, the brain is 75% water and the lungs are nearly 90% water.

DRINK WATER AND PERFORM

Most athletes drink polluted water *(according to research and findings)* thereby polluting muscles, glands and organs, including the brain. The fact is that, the quality of the water they drink has a direct effect *(positive or negative)* on their performance at every stage. Again, it is important to bear in mind that even a low level of pollution will disrupt your beautiful training and performance.

At this level of conviction, I can say that it will always be advantageous for athletes in particular to bear in mind that water is the most important nutrient that they cannot afford to neglect, and it can mean the difference between 100% and 45% performance.

To be candid, 1 was among the first to accept the fact that most athletes do not drink enough water; instead they drink diet sodas, coffee, tea or artificial soft drinks. I am also sure that there is no doubt that athletes must replace lost water constantly. Even a tiny shortage of body fluid will definitely disrupt the body's biomechanical cycles and this is not a healthy path towards becoming a champion.

Note: Dehydrate a muscle by only 2% and you lose 20% in speed and 35% in contractile strength and endurance.

Many of the feelings of fatigue and premature weakness during exercise are as a result of water loss. Do not replace water with coffee, tea and soft drinks; enjoy your beverages in moderation as they may indirectly cause the body to excrete minerals like sodium, potassium or calcium.

During training and competitions, some athletes usually reduce the amount of water they consume because they feel heavy and conclude that their body system *"holds too much water"*. I would strongly refute this idea since what they fail to realise is that the less water they drink, the more their body wants to hold on to every single drop it has in its possession.

My advice is simple and direct; drink whatever water is necessary to comfortably enjoy your meal and drink additional water between meals throughout the day in order to stay hydrated. If for any reason you feel thirsty, please drink water right away, as this will be absorbed quickly and help to avoid dehydration. Dehydration is a condition that will adversely affect the digestion of food, transportation of nutrients and gases, joint lubrication and the regulation of the body temperature.

In a well balanced diet and under normal conditions, dehydration should not be a problem.

Note: - Nothing is better for your health and vitality than the pure, tasteless and good old fashioned water!

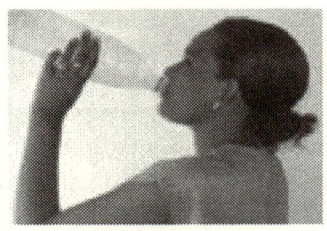

Drinking water before, during and after exercises is crucial

Ironically, even when training moderately in a temperate climate, your body system will still lose one litre of water a day to breathing, sweat and urine. For those athletes that usually train hard in hot weather, there is a tendency that they will lose up to two to three litres of water every 1 to 2 hours. As you can see, the body needs a constant supply of hydration irrespective of any environmental condition or situation in which you are training at any point in time.

At all levels of training *(before, during and after),* make sure that the total intake of water should balance the total output. Should the temperature be high or the exercise you are involved in is strenuous, then additional water should then be taken to make up the body's deficit. If for any reason you do not adequately replace this loss of fluid, then it is your health, vitality and overall performance that will dramatically suffer.

Note: Research reveals that an adequate water intake will generally promote a rapid recovery and thereby enhance glycogen replenishment.

CRAMP AND WATER CONNECTION

Frequently during sports competitions or championships, an athlete will grab his calf and thigh and start screaming in agony - Cramp! Cramp!! Cramp!!!. In most cases what really occurs is a *"painful spasmodic involuntary contraction"* of skeletal muscle that takes place during or immediately after muscular exercise. Before the problem is recognised and probably identified, the athlete is out of the contest and all the hard training and huge amount of money spent on diet, supplements and equipment quickly comes to his mind which can intensify the pain further.

Athletes, coaches and the officiating officials often do not recognise the contributing factors such as:

- Dehydration

- Lack of flexibility

- Lack of minerals such as Calcium, magnesium and iron

- Imbalance of electrolytes such as sodium and potassium

- Muscle fatigue

- Unfavourable temperature (overheating)

- Over stretching of the muscle tissue

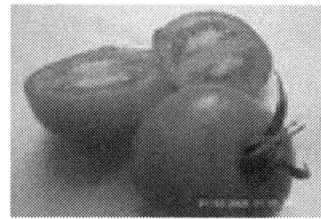

Tomatoes are rich in vitamins (vitamin C) and minerals (calcium)

As you can all see, there are a combination of factors which may actually give rise to most muscle induced cramp as opposed to the idea that only dehydration or the shortage of water in the body should be held responsible for this unforeseen circumstance. Also, from wide scale experience, I believe that knowing this much should help athletes to overcome this regular and often re-occurring predicament.

The factors influencing exercise and associated muscle cramps are complicated and involve the following:

- Central (brain and spinal cord)

- Peripheral (12 pairs of cranial nerves and 312 pairs of spinal nerves) nervous systems,

- Muscle cells (actins and myosin)

Note: Muscles most prone to cramping are those crossing two joints during exercise, which involves the gastrocnemous and hamstring.

Cramp prevention (CP)

Preventative measures are as follows and are the proven solutions to muscle cramps:-

- Proper and effective stretching before training and competition will be of immense benefit

- Stretching vulnerable areas such as the hamstrings, hips, lower back, the gastrocnemous and the soleus can effectively reduce exercise associated muscle cramp *(EAMC)*

- Balanced diet and nutrition can prevent the occurrence of exercise associated muscle cramp *(EAMC)*

- An adequate level of hydration

- Stable electrolyte balance

- Adequate recuperation and restoration of the muscle fibre.

Chapter Seven
FOOD SUPPLEMENTATION FORTIFICATION AND ENRICHMENT.

At no time have I been a major advocate, or have recommended the systematic misuse and abuse of food supplements to competing athletes in the way many physical and health educators may do. I and my colleagues carry out our own research and since we are not paid to endorse any company products, we feel that we can pass on unbiased information and will continue to do so.

Note: - The common argument that supplements will encourage athletes to ignore good nutrition simply does not hold water, especially among those who eat a balanced diet.

Of more importance to me is that many hard training athletes on low – calorie diets could become deficient in many areas of nutrition. This is simply due to much conflicting information in the market place. Though supplements are important, natural food sources will provide all the necessary requirements needed for training, recovery, growth and energy. Indeed, supplements cannot perform any magic if the diet is composed of nothing but processed, artificial flavourings and chemical additives.

It is my hope that athletes will take full advantage of the wealth of natural foods available to them and use them as the tools to make their training and recovery operate at 99%.

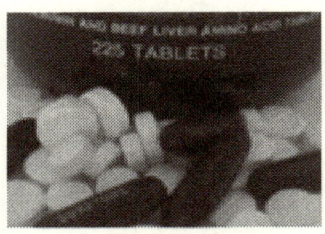

Food supplementation is required by hard training athletes

Note: - The entire necessary nutritional requirements are found in food sources alone. Food and not drugs of any kind should be the basis of the performance of any athlete and should remain so, for both training and achievement purposes.

For years we have seen all variety of advertisements claiming that their magic pill or chemicals will make athletes stronger, bigger, and faster in only 7 days! Food fortification and enrichment have indeed been the *"magic - words"*. Obviously, many if not all athletes are confused about the relative value of some food sources, as most cannot tell a valuable food from one that may be of no benefit whatsoever. Many athletes have suffered and in fact gained nothing from supplements except unwanted weight, illness such as sinus problems, catarrh, increased mucus, blocked mucus membranes, stomach upsets, flatulence and much more.

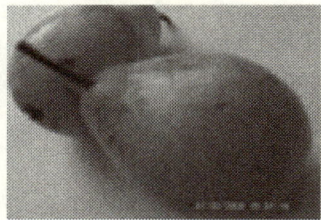

Natural fruit are essential for optimum performance

Athletes commonly use supplements as a sort of insurance policy against missing meals and taking in too few calories. At this juncture, it became necessary as a matter of responsibility and obligation to lead in the area of food supplement education. It is important to speak out about this in order to eliminate the notion that everything over the counter *(OTC)* can help athletes reach their maximum potential.

NOTICE AND GUIDE FOR ATHLETES

Several competing athletes have chosen to join some of these unscrupulous synthetic food manufacturers. Most of them now often claim to have *"the best food supplement under the sun"*. This statement is only for their pocket and not for the benefit of the athlete's health and vitality. What they will never tell athletes is that their whole selling strategy is encapsulated in falsehood, as every advert is only designed for their self interest. On this note, it would be wise and reasonable for all athletes to consult and clarify their food supplementation with experts, before buying or consuming them.

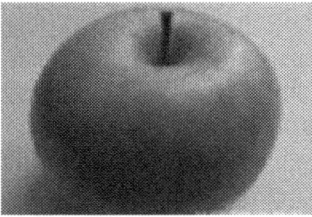

Fresh fruits (Apple) are good for your health and vitality

A simple telephone call to any or relevant anti-drug organisation or dietetic department is the best way to check if a food supplement is suitable and beneficial for your health, vigour and vitality.

Relevant Notice:

- Check expiry dates on products – it makes no sense in buying a product if it has expired.

- Take note of what each supplement that you consume contains - so that you do not consume an excess of the same nutrients, which may result in toxicity and therefore be counter productive.

- Be vigilant – make sure you know both the benefits and the possible side effects of any supplementation

- Avoid *"bogus"* or counterfeit food supplements, which are not easily digested and absorbed smoothly by the body.

- Avoid non-essential - harsh fillers and binders, as used in powder shakes and tablets which are incorporated by some manufacturers. Refrain from purchasing any *"hyped"* up supplement that is labelled as an authentic product.

Furthermore, it is important to explain with full clarity as to how you can effectively avoid buying counterfeit products and how to detect their many selling falsehood strategies.

I will prove my point as follows:

a)   Any attempt to increase the calories per serving size, usually means an increase in the fat content or to include harsh fillers and binders which are of no value to an athlete. The best way to ensure that your food supplement is nutritious and efficient is to take supplements in a serving that could be rapidly absorbed and digested *(280 – 580 calories)*. Also very important to athletes is the composition of the ingredient panel.

b)   50% of the food supplement paraded over the counter *(OTC)*, contains generally *"useless"* formulas. The reason we say *"useless"* is that the body cannot comfortably digest anything more than around 600 calories in one meal. As you should also know, large meals will slow down your metabolism; resulting in you experiencing premature fatigue that will eventually disrupt your training and performance.

c)   Again, 50% of the food supplements available to athletes are made up of low quality nutrients and various mouth watering bogus ingredients. Ensure you buy only a good quality supplement formula that contains a high biological value *(BV)*. The higher the Biological value the more the supplement is absorbed and utilised without waste.

d)   Many nefarious drug manufacturers are now using various sports federations and institutions to deceive and persuade athletes into buying various worthless products. For example, they claim that:-

   • The International Olympic Committee *(IOC)* has cleared their product for the consumption of the athletes.

   • They usually indicate on their product *"IOC allowed"*.

It is important to note that the statement *"IOC allowed"* does not imply that the 10C has officially endorsed their food supplement.

Note: Do not be misled at any level and if in doubt consult a dietician, pharmacist or relevant anti – drug agency.

Stay clear of inexpensive, heavily processed, unprescribed pills and powders. Most are capable and responsible for destroying the future of many competing athletes and occasionally have led to the suspension or an outright ban as a result of their use/misuse/abuse. So do ensure that you get only the best *(authentic)* product when choosing a food supplement.

INCREASING NEED FOR SUPPLEMENTS

Over the past 15 years and more recently it has become clear that daily fortification or enrichment of food with multivitamins and trace elements has been useful at all levels of training and performance, especially for those training hard at National and International championship levels.

Food supplementation has helped to eradicate many performance – threatening problems, and currently there is an increased hope among experts that food supplements will help to ensure a strong and healthier competitive lifestyle for a larger segment of athletes across all sport.

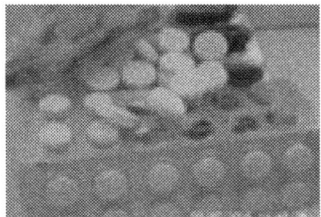

Supplements provides insurance against malnutrition

Note: - *If* you are deficient in nutritious food, recovery from heavy training may be hindered or affected though you may not be aware of it.

In many instances we have talked both about how and what athletes eat, and how they do not eat the right foods in order to provide their entire nutrient requirement. Many athletes are eating poor, fast foods in which nutrients are depleted. More problematic however, are those who find it difficult to take 2 – 3 cooked meals a day. This category of athletes should find it easy to adopt a suitable nutritional supplement, in order to provide the important macro and micronutrients to sustain and maintain high intensity training and muscle growth.

Athletes who are more likely to require supplements are:

- *Athletes with excessive menstrual bleeding.*

- *Athletes taking oral contraceptives*

- *Athletes who consume a diet low in calories (Less than 1,500 calories a day)*

- *Athletes who frequently rely on diets that do not meet their nutritional requirement.*

- *Others are - smokers, those who have a high alcohol intake and those taking diuretics.*

SUPPLEMENTS AS AN INSURANCE POLICY

Food experts may argue endlessly over the precise nutritional requirements to enable intermediate and high level athletes to train hard and compete regularly. One aspect that no one could argue is that exercise increases the loss of vitamins and minerals.

Our findings concluded that whatever sport you are doing, from powerlifting to marathon running, your body breaks down vital nutrients and in particular those reserve stores within the muscle tissue. Failure by an athlete to adequately replenish these vital nutrients will result in reduced recovery and strength, loss of muscle mass, fatigue and burnout which eventually leads to severe injuries to bones, ligaments and tendons. It may also result in permanent damage to organs in the body system.

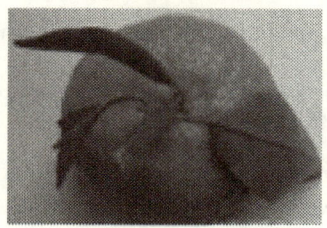

Fresh orange, can refresh and revitalise athletes

Athletes who take supplements especially those of non-pharmaceutical base are more likely to eat a healthy nutrient rich diet. Instead of relying on supplement, they take advantage of supplement as an insurance against any deficiencies in their diet and nutrition.

The benefit derived from food supplements in sport seems undeniable especially when we consider the various research and studies at our disposal, which show clearly that the incidence of vitamin and mineral deficiency among those who relied on diet alone was - *47%* as and only *12%* among those who supplemented.

Chapter Eight
PROPER DIET TO AID RECOVERY

No matter what your determination and aspirations are as an athlete, you will never reach your full potential without a comprehensive diet and sufficient rest. My prime goal in this segment is to make sure that, athletes across all sport truly understand how the body system recuperates from the chemical by-products; produced from muscle contraction especially during training and competitions.

Notes: - The accumulation of excess lactic acid over a long period of time can be detrimental, since these chemicals cause biological phenomena such as muscular soreness.

During the muscular and vascular contractility that usually accompanies training or competitions, by-products such as excess lactic acid accumulate from the combustion of foodstuffs and can prove problematic. Normally, the process of energy release is a remarkably healthy process, but what is not healthy for athletes is the *"chemical process"*. This could be harmful to the anatomical and physiological composition of the body, especially if it is deficient in the nutrients needed to flush them out of the system in an efficient process.

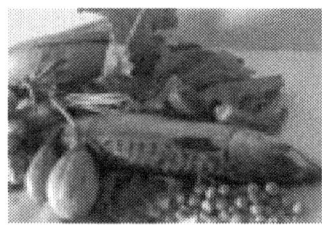

Balanced diet will help in building a strong healthy lifestyle

The most important ingredient in muscular recovery is nutrition. If your nutritional intake is lacking in protein, carbohydrates, vitamins, minerals and water then –

- The body is going to be somewhat limited in its ability to recover effectively

- The proper functioning of organs and tissues that furnish the body with needed energy will be impaired.

Also to be noted is that not all muscles recover at the same rate, larger muscles require a longer period of time to recover while the small muscle parts take a lesser period of time to undergo recovery. A simple description of how athletes eat, train and recuperate could be well understood by using the analogy of logs burning in a fireplace:

- The log is an example of (food) which is ingested into the body.

- The flame represents the energy generated by muscles to perform a specific task (concentric and eccentric activities).

Note: The faster you can remove free radicals from the system, the faster your recovery from intense training.

When logs burn in a fireplace whether mildly or intensely, smoke ascends into the atmosphere and ashes the (by-product) accumulate in the fireplace. Therefore you should know that:-

- The more the logs you burn in the fireplace - the more ashes accumulate in the fireplace

At a certain stage the fireplace will definitely need to be cleaned out so as not to occlude or interfere with the process at which the fire burns fresh logs. I strongly believe without any doubt, that the same process applies to your body system on a daily basis otherwise your muscles will refuse to work efficiently, and will not receive sufficient energy in order to perform additional work.

It should be of no surprise to many athletes that their muscles recover while they are sleeping or relaxing, and that athletes from varying sports backgrounds require different amounts of sleep. If your sleep is interrupted for any reason, it will not leave you feeling rested and it is likely therefore that your body will not have recovered. Athletes at every level of training and competition need a minimum and maximum of 8 – 9 hours sleep every night.

At this stage it should be clear that the best form of relaxation will definitely come from sleep that involves the Rapid Eye Movement, *(REM)*. This is the period of time during sleep when the process of recuperation and restoration takes place in a circular form to build, re-build and repair muscle tissues. However, the fact is that all of this will simply be impossible without a balanced and nutritious diet.

Note: - **Every training programme you directly or indirectly involve yourself in requires calories to be burnt for fuel.**

SLEEP AND DIET - FOR OPTIMUM PERFORMANCE

Intense training and poor diet could place more demand on your resting and relaxation ability which could eventually wreck your performance. This will likely lead you to over-training which is often associated with decreased performance, muscle weakness and soreness, psychological depression, lack of energy and motivation. The end result may be giving up your sports dreams and aspirations. So, if you deprive your body system of a balanced diet, optimum recovery from sleep and relaxation, then you are bound to experience a frequent feeling of weariness and the mal-functioning of some of the body's physiological systems.

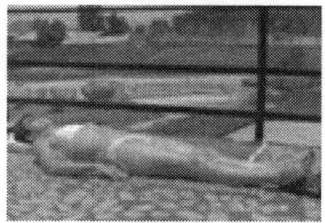

Proper relaxation is the key to optimum recovery

Athletes should always consume a balanced diet so that they can keep their body in a constant supply of adequate energy and vitality. Complete restoration usually involves significant time and resources but can actually reduce the effect of heavy training. On the other hand, regular or frequent incomplete restoration leads to chronic exhaustion, a diminished training effect and an accumulation of functional disturbances in the body which may lead to long term health and physical problems.

Ironically, it is during sleep and not during training that your body releases growth hormones (GH). Again, if you can not wake up in the morning without an alarm clock, definitely you are not getting enough sleep and invariably your training and performance will suffer considerably.

NOTE: - Fatigue is a defence mechanism of the body and it reminds you of the extreme functional and biochemical changes that occur when work is done

GATEWAY TO PROPER RELAXATION

- *Do not take to sedatives as a way to gain proper relaxation*

- *Avoid caffeine containing soft drinks especially during the evening to avoid insomnia*

- *Do not go to bed either hungry, dehydrated or too full*

- *Avoid taking to drugs at every point in time to normalise situations. For example - to stimulate appetite, recuperation, restoration and relaxation*

- *Refrain from alcohol, even if a few glasses can send you to go to bed easily, but you are more likely to wake up in the middle of the night and have trouble getting back to sleep. Not to mention the hangover effect the following day!*

- *Try not to have daytime naps if you are one of those who can not easily sleep at night*

- *Pay attention to your pillow – your neck and head needs a good support, but too thick a pillow can literally be a pain in the neck!*

- *A durable, comfortable mattress is crucial to proper relaxation; purchase a new mattress if the need arises without excitation.*

- *Stress and worries are a common factor in sleeplessness. Always try your best and remain focused.*

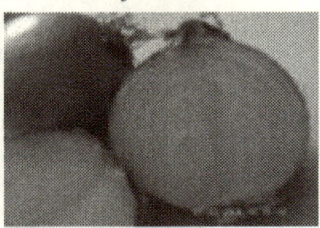

Onions are examples of minerals vital for good living

In conclusion, along with diet and nutrition comes training and relaxation which are the essence of sport. So always choose your food and mode of recuperation, restoration and relaxation wisely, because your lifestyle will eventually determine what you can become in sport.

Chapter Nine
QUESTIONS AND FEEDBACK

WHAT DIET TRULY STANDS FOR!

QUESTION:

I strongly believe that "dieting," means deprivation, hunger, misery and more self- sacrifice than anyone can endure. Please, can you please confirm or dispute this notion?

BD VERSUS BD FEEDBACK:

A diet should not be that way if you eat sensibly and in fact it would be wise at this stage to properly define diet as *"eating behaviour"*.

Sports medicine specialists and nutritionists know that balanced diets are essential for the optimal functioning of body systems such as:–

- Muscle contractions

- Nerve impulses,

- Bone structure formation

- Energy metabolism

- Fluid balance and more.

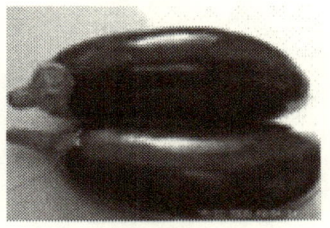

Aubergines are natural, fresh and without any preservatives

Experts also state that: *"No day-to-day activities rely more on good diet and nutrition than sport"*- without which so many athletes would not become champions. Competitive athletes like yourself should know that it is always wise and reasonable to be more compliant with your dietary regimen, in order for your health and vitality to enjoy the subsequent benefits of a lifestyle predicated on sensible eating pattern.

- *You must not skip meals*

- *Your food should be directly proportional to the energy you expend during training.*

- *Eat a good breakfast, lunch and dinner at regular intervals.*

Note: Most athletes hate diets or find them difficult to maintain and the more they hate this proper eating habit, the more their goals suffer and sometimes disintegrate.

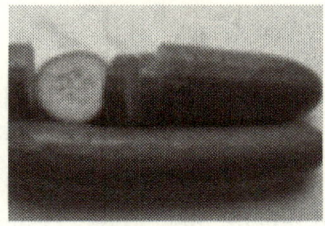

Cucumbers are natural and contain no chemical additives

Contradiction is abundant at every level of diet and nutrition which may serve to confuse both you and others. Never the less, you must ensure that your body is replenished regularly and should you need a *low glycemic index content snack* in between meals, go for any natural source with a high nutrient content.

This will enable you to maintain a strong healthy and solid performance in your chosen field of sport. Finally, if you abide by the simple rules of eating plenty of fresh fruit and vegetables, less fatty meat and fish, this regimen will enable you to continue enjoying the occasional treat such as cheese cake, burger, ice cream and so on.

NUTRITION FOR THOUGHT

QUESTION:

Most athletes including myself stick to a particular food on a daily basis. Although, most simply refer to it as "our favourites", what are the benefits and disadvantages of this monotonous dietary routine?

BD VERSUS BD FEEDBACK:

This idea does not and will not make sense at any level, because if you constantly eat the same meal day after day for any particular reason best known to you, then it will be virtually impossible for you to maintain an adequate intake of nutrients that will support the efficient recovery and growth needed for optimal performance.

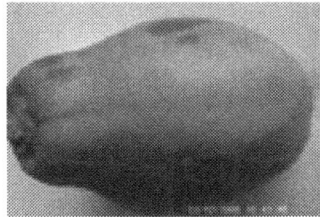

Pawpaw provides wide range of vitamins and minerals

Past experience indicates that persuading athletes to eat sensibly can be a major problem, as many probably pick up *"bad eating habits"* from fellow athletes, some coaches and the media. The big question here is why should you operate at 75% if you can operate at 99%? Also as a serious minded and aspiring athlete, if you are still in the habit of eating the same food day after day, then you may have to be content with *"never becoming a champion in your lifetime"*!

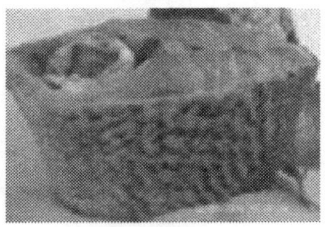

Fish is very rich in iron and at its best when eaten fresh

Clearly many athletes are notorious for poor eating habits, but the simple truth is *"No balanced diet = No balanced performance"*. My conclusion is simple and direct, and that is to say that any athlete who eats one particular food on a daily basis with lack of variety *(which is the spice of vigour and longevity!)*, will only be depriving himself the tools needed to develop the engine necessary to drive him to the position of a champion.

THE FRESHER THE BETTER

QUESTION:

Some athletes always try to eat natural food as frequently as possible, with the added hope that it will provide the desired advantage. I would appreciate an explanation, especially in relation to sports performance.

BD VERSUS BD FEEDBACK:

Athletes should always avoid processed and refined foods whenever possible, instead should always eat fresh foods. They must also ensure that only essential nutrients are put into the body system. Processed foods are typically high in added fat, often hidden sugar, sodium and other chemical additives. Most processed foods, if not all, have their vitamins and minerals eroded during processing and packaging.

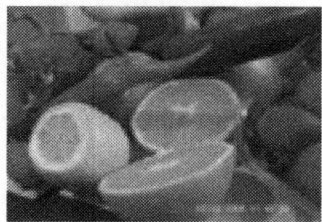

The fresher the food the better for the athletes

Optimal performance in sport requires less sodium, less refinement, less junk and more of the natural components of diet and nutrition. Natural foods, such as vegetables and fruit juices are preferable to soft carbonated drinks; especially if you can *"juice"* fresh fruits at home for immediate consumption, as opposed to the commercial type that have been heavily processed, bottled or canned and then distributed through various mediums from one country or continent to another.

It is my hope that athletes know that even light heating or cooking during processing, manufacturing and packaging of food can result in loss or damage to vitamins, mineral and trace elements. The onus is on athletes to always - as a matter of priority, to ensure that his/her diet and overall nutritional intake is fresh and retains its essential nutrients. This is an indication that the body system is 99% maintained on natural, unprocessed and nutrient enriched food.

Endeavour to always scrutinise food stuffs before you purchase them, also reading labels on food items is good and essential. Athletes are not at all nutritionally aware and may think they are getting exactly what is required for optimum performance. Various documented facts have proved to us of late that even a product that is carefully packaged to look wholesome from every angle, may have been subjected to high temperatures or other detrimental processing procedures.

The bottom line is, natural or raw foods usually have most of their original nutrient contents intact with fewer undesirable additives.

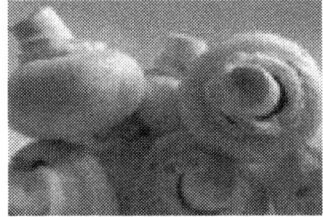

Mushrooms are rich in essential vitamins

MUCH TO LEARN ABOUT METABOLISM

QUESTION:

What is metabolism and how does it benefit my performance, enhance my health, vitality and overall well being?

BD VERSUS BD FEEDBACK:

Metabolism refers to the whole range of chemical and physiological processes by which a living organisms produce energy to maintain and sustain vital functions, such as the replacement of cells, the ability to recuperate and promote muscle development. Every athlete must know that without these fundamental activities taking place efficiently and consistently within the body system, their efforts in the gym or on track will still be rendered useless. This is irrespective of any sophisticated or proven technique ever invented by scientists and coaches that they may adopt. With the added hope of achieving their goal in sport.

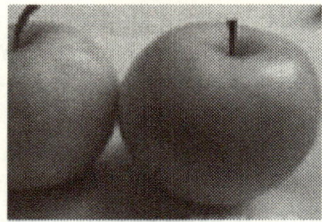

Apples are a good source of B vitamin (Water soluble) and good for the metabolism

I am confident that if athletes take time to study comprehensively and understand how metabolism functions, they will be surprised at how easier champions are made without having to use/misuse/abuse any performance enhancing poison.

The bottom line is simple and direct, whatever your sport at least a sound knowledge of your metabolic rate puts you in control of your training, recuperative and restoration ability, therefore ensuring that your performance continues to progress at a reasonable pace.

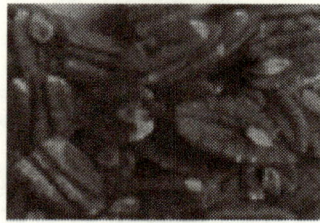

Pecan nut kennels are rich in fibre and aids metabolism

Again, this understanding will enable you to determine how your body system uses and disposes what you consume and will help you to prevent becoming overweight and obese, whilst simultaneously fuelling your energy levels and muscles to a higher level of performance..

WHEN IS BEVERAGE NOT REQUIRED

QUESTION:

Many athletes now use coffee and some herbal tea to legally enhance their performance and as fluid replacement therapy. Most often claim it is a beverage and part and parcel of a healthy sports diet.

I would appreciate an explanation as to what is the correlation between (diet and nutrition) and (coffee and tea) in relation to sports performance.

BD VERSUS BD FEEDBACK:

First and foremost, food is a substance which when digested and absorbed into the body system through the alimentary tract will subsequently - via the bloodstream be capable of supplying the body with calories. From this, heat is generated to form the energy needed to train and compete. This aids growth generally and provides the ability to repair its worn out tissues. Here it should be noted that neither "tea nor coffee" in any way, fulfil any of these obligations and therefore cannot be classified as foods.

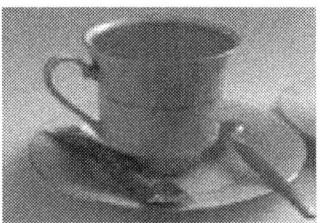

Water provides good health - not tea, coffee or either beverages

Both tea and coffee contain the *"alkaloid caffeine"*. Caffeine is a stimulant and can be easily misused and abused by unscrupulous athletes, nevertheless this does not mean that coffee and tea have no value in the daily diet. Caffeine in many instances:-

- Abolishes the sense of fatigue

- Causes insomnia in most people

- It increases the ability for mental and physical work

Over indulgence or continuous use/misuse/abuse of coffee and tea in any form may lead to an increased and abnormal excitability of the nervous systems.

Note: Never combine coffee, herbal tea, strong chocolate or cola with good diet, as it will render nutritious food useless.

RESEARCH – CAFFEINE AND ADRENALINE

When adrenaline is naturally released into the blood stream during competition, it sets in motion a process known as the *"fight or flight response"*. It produces physiological effects, such as elevated heart rate and increases blood pressure that sets you up for action. This response, even as natural as it is can cause:-

- Heart rhythm disturbance

- Angina *(Chest pain or discomfort that occurs when your heart muscle does not get enough blood).*

- Chronically elevated blood pressure

Now imagine an artificial stimulant and diuretic like coffee and tea being introduced to further stimulate the system to over – produce adrenaline to abnormal levels, such practices will produce undesirable effects on the health and the overall well being of the user/misuse/abuser.

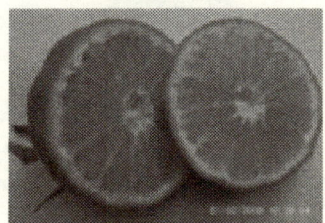

Orange instead of tea or coffee after an intense workout is preferable

Notes the following;-

i)   *Caffeine is a diuretic. It acts directly on the kidneys and increases the output of urine. Do not use cola, coffee or herbal tea to replace lost fluid. Make sure you get 3-4 litres of fresh water each day.*

ii)   *Caffeine acts upon the nerve centres that control the lungs and heart, it also acts on both respiratory and cardiac muscles which* can stimulate or over-stimulate these organs depending on its availability and the amount of intake by an individual.

iii)   *Can aggravate conditions, such as:-*

- *Gastric and duodenal ulcer*

- *Gastritis*

Note*:* Tea and coffee should be avoided or forbidden altogether - before, during or after training.

ALCOHOL - TO DRINK OR NOT TO DRINK

QUESTION:

Athletes are under pressure not to experiment with alcohol of any kind and are now drinking non – alcoholic drinks as a alternative. It would be nice if an explanation can be given as to the effect of alcohol and if there is any benefit in choosing non-alcoholic drinks.

BD VERSUS BD FEEDBACK:

To be candid, I do not know of anything that is so good about non-alcoholic beer, other than the lack of alcohol. Non-alcoholic drinks have only one third or one half the calories of regular alcohol. Both alcohol and non-alcohol beverages are basically carbohydrates with a small amount of mineral and B vitamins.

Alcohol and non-alcoholic drinks should not be counted as fluid replacements - they are not and will never be. Instead they indirectly increase your need for fluid. This is part of the reason why hard training athletes especially in hot climates must regularly replace body fluid which is lost through perspiration with plain, clean water and not alcohol or non-alcoholic drinks under any guise.

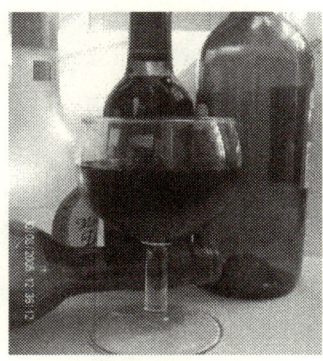

Alcohol is not a good friend of a champion or champion to be

To achieve progress at any level of sport requires discipline, dedication and will power! That is why you must refrain and abstain from abusing your body with alcohol for the following reasons:

i)   *Alcohol decreases the ability to reason properly and exaggerates emotion. Athletes who consume alcohol in and around the sports environment can get unruly and often make complete fools of themselves before, during and after a competition.*

ii)   *Alcohol or the hangover effect of alcohol often leads to arguments with judges, officiating officials and fellow athletes, which can in turn lead to increased aggression, damage to equipment and facilities. This unruly behaviour often results in a suspension, ban or worse still to possible arrest.*

iii)   *Alcohol boosts your emotions unnecessarily and lowers your guard, and as a result you are much more likely to engage in reckless behaviour which can put sport into a state of disrepute.*

iv)   *During training and championships, the athlete "binger" does not feel motivated to take part in any exercise routine. Even if he does exercise at all he is likely to be less focused and less likely to reach any effective level of training..*

v)   *Alcohol lowers testosterone for up to 72 hours and increases oestrogen levels. If you really want to achieve the best from your training and competitions, then you must abstain from alcohol.*

Notes: - The carcinogen producing substance in alcohol called nitrosamine which is present in most beers is thought to be a possible culprit in the increased prevalence of rectal cancer among heavy beer drinkers.

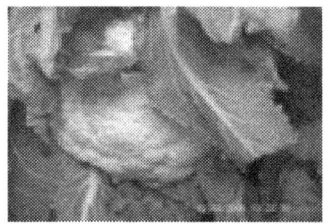

Cauliflower is highly rich in vitamins and minerals

Finally, alcohol is a useless nutrient and gets stored easily as fat because of the high calorific content. Drinkers may also require more minerals, fat soluble vitamins and B vitamins.

Alcohol has the potential at every level to destroy lives, aspiration, focus and your overall well being.

CIGARETTE -- SMOKING FOR WEIGHT LOSS

QUESTION:

Some overweight athletes often claim that cigarette smoking is part of their weight loss dietary regimen. Frankly speaking, how can smoke help athletes to lose weight?

BD VERSUS BD FEEDBACK:

In the first instance smoking acts as an appetite suppressor and of equal significance is the fact that cigarette smoking raises the need for vitamin B_2 *(Riboflavin)* and vitamin C *(Ascorbic acid)* amongst others. Finally, the image of the smoker brings to mind lung cancer, also extensive research shows that smoking causes irreversible damage to the cardiovascular system - examples are arteries, veins, lungs and to the heart itself.

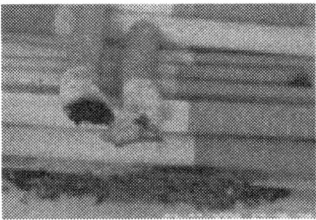

Cigarettes is an enemy of the cardiovascular and respiratory systems

Note: - Without getting too complex, you should eat at least one fruit and one vegetable high in Vitamin C every day.

As a smoker, this will provide an ample supply of B Vitamins. However, this is not a licence to smoke!

Ironically, smokers often use the desire to remain thin or to lose weight as an excuse for their bad habit. Recent findings show that smoking might influence fat production in the abdomen rather than the hips. This predisposes the person to an increased risk of:-

- Heart disease
- Emphysema
- Strokes
- Diabetes

It would be beneficial for athletes to know that *(side stream smoke)* which is the smoke from the burning end of a cigarette actually contains a higher concentration of harmful compounds than smoke inhaled directly *(main stream smoke)* by the smoker. Again side stream smoke has:-

- Twice as much *tar and nicotine*
- Three times as much *carbon monoxide*

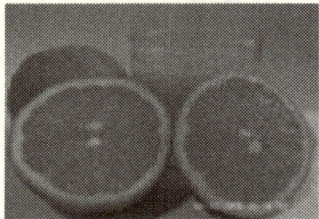

Fresh orange (juiced) will definitely revitalise you

Most of the smoke in a room is side stream. Non smokers suffer in smoke filled air. Inhalation of carbon monoxide depletes oxygen in the blood by displacing oxygen in the red blood cells. Again, it is important to note that oxygen utilisation by the body can influence a good or a bad performance.

Note: Oxygen – depleted level in the blood can impact significantly on the heart and the overall well being.

Athletes at all levels should know that carbon monoxide can cause acute breathing difficulties and asthma like symptoms which will invariably affect performance and result in weakness and fatigue

NEVER BEEN SCIENTIFICALLY PROVEN?

QUESTION:

The new slogans – "it has never been scientifically proven" has made it to be so difficult to restore the significance of good diet and nutrition among athletes. I hope you would dispel this naïve perception.

BD VERSUS BD FEEDBACK:

The key word here is what "proven" means to the athletes. Typical examples are:

i)   *It has not been proven that a balanced diet is the key to a sustainable long healthy life.*

ii)   *It has not been proven that anabolic-androgenic steroids cause any health problems.*

iii)   *It has not been proven that a balanced diet is better than banned drugs.*

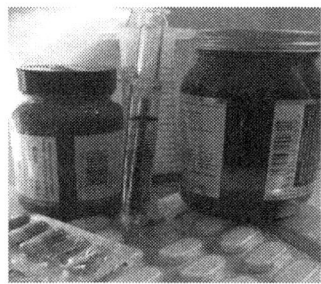

It is quite ridiculous that some athletes still believe that anabolic – androgenic steroids cause no health problems

Unfortunately this notorious perception has made it so difficult for many athletes to distinguish between *"hype and hope"*, and what is more alarming is the profound discouraging attitude of some athletes towards a sensible eating behaviour.

Most dangerous of all is the misleading, dedicated campaign directed at those trying to do what is right and proper for their own health, sport as a whole and that of society at large.

As a result of this, many think tanks are now trying to figure out exactly what can be done to effectively reduce the nutritional disadvantages experienced by athletes over the years, also to propel the body with a whole range of proven effective dietary and nutritional guidelines. Along this line of action, the genuine effort taken by more liberal minded athletes regarding diet and nutrition has proved to be the only viable option to ensure a proven healthy future performance

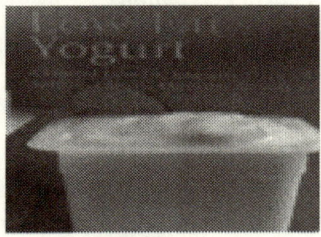

It has been scientifically proven that yogurt provides a good source of protein

Health and fitness is all about choices, for some making the right choice is easy because they choose to move in the right direction. On the other hand there are those who travel with the wrong group who deliberately lead them down the wrong and often painful road of no return. In some cases individuals travel alone without any assistance and still often make the wrong choices, simply because they lack awareness, proper nurturing and grooming within the sport arena.

It is my hope that every serious minded athlete will ignore this misconception– *"it has never been scientifically proven"* and use facts and verifiable scientific findings to shock their body into an effective and prosperous sports career.

Reference

Maclean, D.A. T; E Graham and B.Saltin. Branched –chain amino acids augment ammonia metabolism while alternating protein breakdown during exercise, American Journal of Physiology 267; E1010 – E1022 1994.

Costill D.L. Miller. JM. Nutrition for endurance sports; Carbohydrate and fluid balance: International journal of sports medicine 112-14.1980.

Wechster. H. et al, correlates of college student binge drinking AMERICA JOURNAL OF PUBLIC HEALTH 85-921-926, 1995.

Okunleff p. interactions between ascorbic acid and the radiation of bone marrow, skin and tumor; 12815-35.

Hem-ufit Magazin Alli-Balogun Alli-Baba 1996/97 Health, muscle and fitness information and advocate

Cade, R et' al. Effects of phosphate loading on 2, 3 diphosphoglycerate and maximum oxygen uptake. Medicine and science in sports and exercise 16. 263-268.1994.

Noakes, T.D. The hyponatremia of exercise. International journal of sports nutrition 2(3). 205-228.1992

Schwelinus MP Derman.E.W. Noakes.TP. Aetiology of skeletal muscle cramp during exercise, a novel hypothesis. Journal of sports science 15(3). 277-285.

Beatley S. Exercise induced muscle cramp. Mechanism and management. Sports medicine 21(6). 409-420. 1992.

Alli-Balogun Alli-Baba 2003 Drugs and Sports-a losing proposition. Anti-Drugs (Prohibited and banned drugs) Rules and regulation

McArdle, WD, Karch, Fl, Katch, VL sports AND exercise nutrition. Philadelphia: Lippincott Williams AND Wilkins, 1999.

Whitney, E.N, Rolfes, S.R. Understanding nutrition (7TH Ed). Minneapolis/ St. Paul: West publishingco.1996.

Index

About the Author

He is an individual consciously committed to the idea of a sustainable and predictable healthy – lifestyle, in sport as well as in life generally. A former athlete with a wondrous sport and administrative career, who has over the past years published various anti-drug magazines, journals, pamphlets and books.

- A physical and health educator per excellence.
- An advocate of drug –free-sport.
- A consultant to numerous informational and anti-drug agencies in Africa and Europe.
- Coordinator - Parents and Athletes against Drugs in Sports.
- Athlete's representative - Common-wealth games and Africa championship etc

Areas of Specialties (Sports)

- Athletic
- Judo
- Football
- Table tennis
- Karate
- Swimming
- Bodybuilding
- Gymnastic
- Weight lifting

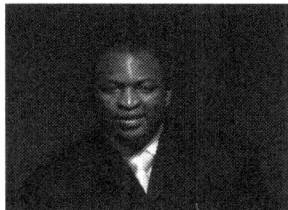

Alli-Balogun Alli- Baba
Co-ordinator
Parents and Athletes against Drugs in Sports
P.A.A.D.S